Biological and Neurobehavioral Studies of Borderline Personality Disorder

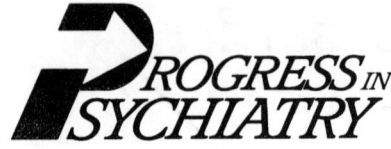

PROGRESS IN PSYCHIATRY

Number 45

David Spiegel, M.D.
Series Editor

Biological and Neurobehavioral Studies of Borderline Personality Disorder

Edited by
Kenneth R. Silk, M.D.

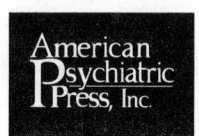

Washington, DC
London, England

Note: The authors have worked to ensure that all information in this book concerning drug dosages, schedules, and routes of administration is accurate as of the time of publication and consistent with standards set by the U.S. Food and Drug Administration and the general medical community. As medical research and practice advance, however, therapeutic standards may change. For this reason and because human and mechanical errors sometimes occur, we recommend that readers follow the advice of a physician who is directly involved in their care or in the care of a member of their family.

Books published by the American Psychiatric Press, Inc., represent the views and opinions of the individual authors and do not necessarily represent the policies and opinions of the Press or the American Psychiatric Association.

Copyright © 1994 American Psychiatric Press, Inc.

ALL RIGHTS RESERVED

Manufactured in the United States of America on acid-free paper

First Edition   97 96 95 94   4 3 2 1

American Psychiatric Press, Inc.
1400 K Street, N.W., Washington, DC 20005

Library of Congress Cataloging-in-Publication Data
Biological and neurobehavioral studies of borderline personality disorder / edited by Kenneth R. Silk. — 1st ed.
    p. cm. — (Progress in psychiatry series ; #45)
  Includes bibliographical references and index.
  ISBN 0-88048-480-2
  1. Borderline personality disorder—Pathophysiology.
  2. Borderline personality disorder—Chemotherapy.
  I. Silk, Kenneth R., 1944- . II. Series.
  [DNLM: 1. Borderline Personality Disorder.
  2. Brain—physiopathology. 3. Neuropsychology—methods.
  W1 PR6781 no.45 1994 / WM 190 B615 1994]
  RC569.5.B67B56 1994
  616.85'85207—dc20
  DNLM/DLC   93-44846
  for Library of Congress   CIP

British Library Cataloguing in Publication Data
A CIP record is available from the British Library.

Contents

Contributors   vii

Introduction: From First- to Second-Generation Biological Studies of Borderline Personality Disorder   xvii
   Kenneth R. Silk, M.D.

1   Impulsivity in Borderline Personality Disorder   1
   Robert van Reekum, M.D., F.R.C.P.C.
   Paul S. Links, M.D., F.R.C.P.C.
   Cecilia Fedorov, R.N.

2   Impulsivity and Serotonin in Borderline Personality Disorder   23
   Marie-Louise deVegvar, M.D.
   Larry J. Siever, M.D.
   Robert L. Trestman, M.D., Ph.D.

3   The Cholinergic and Noradrenergic Neurotransmitter Systems and Affective Instability in Borderline Personality Disorder   41
   Bonnie Jean Steinberg, M.D.
   Robert L. Trestman, M.D., Ph.D.
   Larry J. Siever, M.D.

4   Peripheral Catecholamine Alterations in Borderline Personality Disorder   63
   Rachel Yehuda, Ph.D.
   Steven M. Southwick, M.D.
   Bruce D. Perry, M.D., Ph.D.
   Earl L. Giller, M.D., Ph.D.

5 Borderline Personality Disorder and the Anxiety
   Disorders   91
   Kenneth R. Silk, M.D.
   JoAnn Goodson, B.S.N., M.P.H.
   Jane Benjamin, Ph.D.
   Naomi E. Lohr, Ph.D.

6 Brain Imaging in Personality Disorders   109
   Peter F. Goyer, M.D.
   P. Eric Konicki, M.D.
   S. Charles Schulz, M.D.

7 Neuropsychological Testing Results in Borderline
   Personality Disorder   127
   Kathleen M. O'Leary, M.S.W.
   Rex William Cowdry, M.D.

8 Neurological Dysfunction in Borderline Patients
   and Axis II Control Subjects   159
   Mary C. Zanarini, Ed.D.
   Catherine R. Kimble, M.D.
   Amy A. Williams, B.S.

9 Early Abuse, Limbic System Dysfunction, and
   Borderline Personality Disorder   177
   Martin H. Teicher, M.D., Ph.D.
   Yutaka Ito, M.D., Ph.D.
   Carol A. Glod, R.N., M.S., C.S.
   Fred Schiffer, M.D.
   Harris A. Gelbard, M.D., Ph.D.

10 "Quo Vademus?"—New Directions in Borderline
   Personality Disorder Research   209
   Rex William Cowdry, M.D.

11 Implications of Biological Research for Clinical
   Work With Borderline Patients   227
   Kenneth R. Silk, M.D.

   Index   241

Contributors

Jane Benjamin, Ph.D.
Clinical Psychologist, Ann Arbor, Michigan

Rex William Cowdry, M.D.
Acting Deputy Director, National Institute of Mental Health, Rockville, MD

Marie-Louise deVegvar, M.D.
Instructor, Department of Psychiatry, Mount Sinai School of Medicine, New York, New York; Bronx Veterans Affairs Medical Center, Bronx, New York

Cecilia Fedorov, R.N.
Department of Psychiatry, McMaster University, Hamilton, Ontario, Canada

Harris A. Gelbard, M.D., Ph.D.
Assistant Professor of Neurology, University of Rochester School of Medicine, Rochester, New York

Earl L. Giller, M.D., Ph.D.
Associate Director, CNS Research, Pfizer Company, Groton, Connecticut

Carol A. Glod, R.N., M.S., C.S.
Clinical Nurse Specialist, Department of Psychiatry, Harvard Medical School, Boston, Massachusetts; Developmental Biopsychiatry Research Program, McLean Hospital, Belmont, Massachusetts

JoAnn Goodson R.N., M.P.H.
Research Nurse, Department of Psychiatry, The University of Michigan, Ann Arbor, Michigan

Peter F. Goyer, M.D.
Chief of Staff, Cleveland Veterans Affairs Medical Center, Brecksville, Ohio; Associate Professor of Psychiatry and Radiology, Case Western Reserve University Medical School, Cleveland, Ohio

Yutaka Ito, M.D., Ph.D.
Research Fellow, Department of Psychiatry, Harvard Medical School, Boston, Massachusetts; Developmental Biopsychiatry Research Program, McLean Hospital, Belmont, Massachusetts

Catherine R. Kimble, M.D.
Clinical Fellow, Department of Psychiatry, Harvard Medical School, Boston, Massachusetts; McLean Hospital, Belmont, Massachusetts

P. Eric Konicki, M.D.
Cleveland Veterans Affairs Medical Center, Brecksville, Ohio; Assistant Professor of Psychiatry, Case Western Reserve University Medical School, Cleveland, Ohio

Paul S. Links, M.D., F.R.C.P.C.
Professor, Department of Psychiatry, University of Toronto; Clinical Director, Department of Psychiatry, Wellesley Hospital, Toronto, Ontario, Canada

Naomi E. Lohr, Ph.D.
Assistant Professor, Departments of Psychiatry and Psychology, The University of Michigan, Ann Arbor, Michigan

Kathleen M. O'Leary, M.S.W.
Research Social Worker, National Institute of Mental Health, Neuroscience Center at St. Elizabeths, Washington, DC

Bruce D. Perry, M.D., Ph.D.
Associate Professor of Psychiatry, Pediatrics, and Pharmacology, Baylor College of Medicine, Houston, Texas

Contributors

Fred Schiffer, M.D.
Clinical Instructor in Psychiatry, Harvard Medical School, Boston, Massachusetts; Developmental Biopsychiatry Research Program, McLean Hospital, Belmont, Massachusetts

S. Charles Schulz, M.D.
Professor and Chairman, Department of Psychiatry, Case Western Reserve University Medical School, Cleveland, Ohio

Larry J. Siever, M.D.
Professor of Psychiatry, Mount Sinai School of Medicine, New York, New York; Bronx Veterans Affairs Medical Center, Bronx, New York

Kenneth R. Silk, M.D.
Associate Professor, Associate Chair for Clinical and Administrative Affairs, and Director of Personality Disorders Program; Department of Psychiatry, The University of Michigan, Ann Arbor, Michigan

Steven M. Southwick, M.D.
Associate Professor of Psychiatry, Yale University School of Medicine, New Haven, Connecticut; West Haven Veterans Administration Medical Center, West Haven, Connecticut

Bonnie Jean Steinberg, M.D.
Research Fellow in Psychiatry, Mount Sinai School of Medicine, New York, New York; Bronx Veterans Affairs Medical Center, Bronx, New York

Martin H. Teicher, M.D., Ph.D.
Associate Psychiatrist and Associate Professor of Psychiatry, Harvard Medical School, Boston, Massachusetts; Director, Developmental Biopsychiatry Research Program, McLean Hospital, Belmont, Massachusetts

Robert L. Trestman. M.D., Ph.D.
Assistant Professor of Psychiatry, Mount Sinai School of Medicine, New York, New York; Bronx Veterans Affairs Medical Center, Bronx, New York

Robert van Reekum, M.D., F.R.C.P.C.
Assistant Professor of Psychiatry, McMaster University, Hamilton, Ontario, Canada

Amy A. Williams, B.S.
Senior Clinical Coordinator, McLean Study of Adult Development, McLean Hospital, Belmont, Massachusetts

Rachel Yehuda, Ph.D.
Assistant Professor of Psychiatry, Mount Sinai School of Medicine, New York, New York; Bronx Veterans Affairs Medical Center, Bronx, New York

Mary C. Zanarini, Ed.D.
Assistant Professor of Psychology in Psychiatry, Harvard Medical School, Boston, Massachusetts; Assistant Director, Psychosocial Research Program; Director, McLean Study of Adult Development, McLean Hospital, Belmont, Massachusetts

Introduction to the Progress in Psychiatry Series

The Progress in Psychiatry Series is designed to capture in print the excitement that comes from assembling a diverse group of experts from various locations to examine in detail the newest information about a developing aspect of psychiatry. This series emerged as a collaboration between the American Psychiatric Association's (APA) Scientific Program Committee and the American Psychiatric Press, Inc. Great interest is generated by a number of the symposia presented each year at the APA annual meeting, and we realized that much of the information presented there, carefully assembled by people who are deeply immersed in a given area, would unfortunately not appear together in print. The symposia sessions at the annual meetings provide an unusual opportunity for experts who otherwise might not meet on the same platform to share their diverse viewpoints for a period of 3 hours. Some new themes are repeatedly reinforced and gain credence, whereas in other instances disagreements emerge, enabling the audience and now the reader to reach informed decisions about new directions in the field. The Progress in Psychiatry Series allows us to publish and capture some of the best of the symposia and thus provide an in-depth treatment of specific areas that might not otherwise be presented in broader review formats.

Psychiatry is, by nature, an interface discipline, combining the study of mind and brain, of individual and social environments, of the humane and the scientific. Therefore, progress in the field is rarely linear—it often comes from unexpected sources. Furthermore, new developments emerge from an array of viewpoints that do not necessarily provide immediate agreement but rather expert examination of the issues. We intend to present innovative ideas and data that will enable you, the reader, to participate in this process.

We believe the Progress in Psychiatry Series will provide you with an opportunity to review timely, new information in specific fields of interest as they are developing. We hope you find that the excitement of the presentations is captured in the written word and that this book proves to be informative and enjoyable reading.

David Spiegel, M.D.
Series Editor
Progress in Psychiatry Series

Progress in Psychiatry Series Titles

Biological and Neurobehavioral Studies of Borderline Personality Disorder (#45)
Edited by Kenneth R. Silk, M.D.

Severe Depressive Disorders (#44)
Edited by Leon Grunhaus, M.D., and John F. Greden, M.D.

Clinical Advances in Monoamine Oxidase Inhibitor Therapies (#43)
Edited by Sidney H. Kennedy, M.D., F.R.C.P.C.

Catecholamine Function in Posttraumatic Stress Disorder: Emerging Concepts (#42)
Edited by M. Michele Murburg, M.D.

Management and Treatment of Insanity Acquittees: A Model for the 1990s (#41)
Edited by Joseph D. Bloom, M.D., and Mary H. Williams, M.S., J.D.

Chronic Fatigue and Related Immune Deficiency Syndromes (#40)
Edited by Paul J. Goodnick, M.D., and Nancy G. Klimas, M.D.

Psychopharmacology and Psychobiology of Ethnicity (#39)
Edited by Keh-Ming Lin, M.D., M.P.H., Russell E. Poland, Ph.D., and Gayle Nakasaki, M.S.W.

Electroconvulsive Therapy: From Research to Clinical Practice (#38)
Edited by C. Edward Coffey, M.D.

Multiple Sclerosis: A Neuropsychiatric Disorder (#37)
Edited by Uriel Halbreich, M.D.

Biology of Anxiety Disorders (#36)
Edited by Rudolf Hoehn-Saric, M.D., and
Daniel R. McLeod, Ph.D.

Psychoimmunology Update (#35)
Edited by Jack M. Gorman, M.D., and Robert M. Kertzner, M.D.

Brain Imaging in Affective Disorders (#34)
Edited by Peter Hauser, M.D.

Positron-Emission Tomography in Schizophrenia Research (#33)
Edited by Nora D. Volkow, M.D., and Alfred P. Wolf, Ph.D.

Mental Retardation: Developing Pharmacotherapies (#32)
Edited by John J. Ratey, M.D.

Current Concepts of Somatization: Research and Clinical Perspectives (#31)
Edited by Laurence J. Kirmayer, M.D., F.R.C.P.C., and
James M. Robbins, Ph.D.

Central Nervous System Peptide Mechanisms in Stress and Depression (#30)
Edited by S. Craig Risch, M.D.

Neuropeptides and Psychiatric Disorders (#29)
Edited by Charles B. Nemeroff, M.D., Ph.D.

Negative Schizophrenic Symptoms: Pathophysiology and Clinical Implications (#28)
Edited by John F. Greden, M.D., and Rajiv Tandon, M.D.

The Neuroleptic Nonresponsive Patient: Characterization and Treatment (#27)
Edited by Burt Angrist, M.D., and S. Charles Schulz, M.D.

Combination Pharmacotherapy and Psychotherapy for Depression (#26)
Edited by Donna Manning, M.D., and Allen J. Frances, M.D.

Treatment Strategies for Refractory Depression (#25)
Edited by Steven P. Roose, M.D., and
Alexander H. Glassman, M.D.

Progress in Psychiatry Series Titles

Biological Rhythms, Mood Disorders, Light Therapy, and the Pineal Gland (#24)
Edited by Mohammad Shafii, M.D., and Sharon Lee Shafii, R.N., B.S.N.

Family Environment and Borderline Personality Disorder (#23)
Edited by Paul Skevington Links, M.D.

Amino Acids in Psychiatric Disease (#22)
Edited by Mary Ann Richardson, Ph.D.

Serotonin in Major Psychiatric Disorders (#21)
Edited by Emil F. Coccaro, M.D., and Dennis L. Murphy, M.D.

Personality Disorders: New Perspectives on Diagnostic Validity (#20)
Edited by John M. Oldham, M.D.

Biological Assessment and Treatment of Posttraumatic Stress Disorder (#19)
Edited by Earl L. Giller, Jr., M.D., Ph.D.

Depression in Schizophrenia (#18)
Edited by Lynn E. DeLisi, M.D.

Depression and Families: Impact and Treatment (#17)
Edited by Gabor I. Keitner, M.D.

Depressive Disorders and Immunity (#16)
Edited by Andrew H. Miller, M.D.

Treatment of Tricyclic-Resistant Depression (#15)
Edited by Irl L. Extein, M.D.

Current Approaches to the Prediction of Violence (#14)
Edited by David A. Brizer, M.D., and Martha L. Crowner, M.D.

Tardive Dyskinesia: Biological Mechanisms and Clinical Aspects (#13)
Edited by Marion E. Wolf, M.D., and Aron D. Mosnaim, Ph.D.

Eating Behavior in Eating Disorders (#12)
Edited by B. Timothy Walsh, M.D.

Cerebral Hemisphere Function in Depression (#11)
Edited by Marcel Kinsbourne, M.D.

Psychobiology of Bulimia (#10)
Edited by James I. Hudson, M.D., and
Harrison G. Pope, Jr., M.D.

Psychiatric Pharmacosciences of Children and Adolescents (#9)
Edited by Charles Popper, M.D.

Biopsychosocial Aspects of Bereavement (#8)
Edited by Sidney Zisook, M.D.

Medical Mimics of Psychiatric Disorders (#7)
Edited by Irl Extein, M.D., and Mark S. Gold, M.D.

Can Schizophrenia Be Localized in the Brain? (#6)
Edited by Nancy C. Andreasen, M.D., Ph.D.

The Psychiatric Implications of Menstruation (#5)
Edited by Judith H. Gold, M.D., F.R.C.P.C.

Post-Traumatic Stress Disorder in Children (#4)
Edited by Spencer Eth, M.D., and
Robert S. Pynoos, M.D., M.P.H.

Treatment of Affective Disorders in the Elderly (#3)
Edited by Charles A. Shamoian, M.D.

Premenstrual Syndrome: Current Findings and Future Directions (#2)
Edited by Howard J. Osofsky, M.D., Ph.D., and
Susan J. Blumenthal, M.D.

The Borderline: Current Empirical Research (#1)
Edited by Thomas H. McGlashan, M.D.

Introduction

From First- to Second-Generation Biological Studies of Borderline Personality Disorder

Kenneth R. Silk, M.D.

Ten years ago, this particular book could not have been assembled. Except for a few papers exploring some biological substrates of antisocial personality disorder, there were only isolated studies that investigated biological processes in borderline personality disorder (BPD). Some papers reported pharmacological responsiveness in BPD, and while these reports suggested intrinsic biological processes in BPD, the opinions regarding the underlying biological mechanisms were only inferred. Almost all of these pharmacological studies prior to 1986 consisted of case reports, open clinical trials, or chart reviews.

There is a great demand to know more about the borderline patient. Borderline patients have a reputation for being extremely difficult to treat. They consume far greater amounts of staff and therapist energy than most patients, and they generate strong, complex countertransference reactions. Their repeated suicide threats, self-mutilation, and sudden, impulsive behavior create constant anxiety in their therapists. Borderline patients present with a myriad of clinical problems that span the gamut of Axis I psychopathology (Hoch and Polatin 1949), including affective instability reminiscent of bipolar disorder (Akiskal 1981); transient psychotic or psychotic-like phenomena reminiscent of schizophrenia or posttraumatic stress disorder (Silk et al. 1989;

Zanarini et al. 1990); severe and persistent substance abuse (Dulit et al. 1990); chronic, unremitting depression (Gunderson and Elliott 1985); severe impulsivity (Zanarini 1993); and panic and chronic anxiety states (Kernberg 1975). The difficulties in treatment are compounded by the limited responsivity of borderline patients to both pharmacotherapy and psychotherapy. Borderline patients as a group do not respond well or in any consistent manner to psychopharmacological intervention (Cowdry and Gardner 1988; Gunderson 1986; Soloff et al. 1986b, 1993). Although some patients with BPD respond fairly well to some medications, we have little solid information as to which borderline patient will respond to any specific pharmacological agent (Soloff et al. 1993). Furthermore, borderline patients appear extremely sensitive to side or adverse effects of medications, and they often continue to have breakthrough interpersonal crises despite moderate pharmacological control of some Axis I symptomatology. Borderline patients may complain of boredom, but to us they are never boring.

When psychiatrists are faced with persisting clinical difficulty, there is a need to know more than we do (and perhaps, unfortunately, the wish to do more than we know [Main 1957]). Clinicians and researchers in the field of personality disorders have begun to pay more attention to the domains of neurobiology and pharmacology in the hope that these areas will provide us with clues, if not answers. Recent breakthroughs in the psychopharmacology of schizophrenia with agents such as clozapine and respiridone, advancements in the pharmacological treatment of depression through the use of selective serotonergic reuptake inhibitors, and the pharmacological treatment of obsessive-compulsive disorder as well as panic and anxiety states—once thought to be in the exclusive jurisdiction of the psychodynamic or the behavioral therapist—compel us to turn our intellectual attention toward the biological, neurological, and constitutional factors that might play a role in the etiology and persistence of borderline symptomatology.

Biological research in the area of BPD was a long time coming but it quickly followed the legitimization of the diagnosis of BPD in the psychiatric nomenclature. Prior to DSM-III (American Psychiatric Association 1980), there was no "official" diagnosis of

BPD. Patients with affective lability, unstable interpersonal relationships, very transient psychotic disturbances, and repeated or chronic suicidality and impulsivity have been described for over 50 years in the psychiatric literature. The term *borderline* was first used by Stern in 1938 (Stern 1938). Patients similar to those described by Stern were labeled *ambulatory schizophrenics* by Zilboorg (1941), as "as if" patients by Deutsch (1942), as *pseudoneurotic schizophrenics* by Hoch and Polatin (1949), and as *patients with borderline states* by Knight (1953). These authors believed that the patients they were describing suffered from a milder form or an atypical presentation of schizophrenia.

In the late 1960s, Grinker et al. (1968) conducted the first empirical study of the borderline diagnosis. His group of researchers found four subgroups within the borderline category. One group bordered on the neuroses; another on the psychoses. A third group seemed close to the "as if" patients of Deutsch, and a final group, which was called the *core borderline group,* consisted of patients who acted out, were often depressed, vacillated between overinvolvement and underinvolvement with others, and seemed to lack a consistent self-identity. Grinker and his colleagues were the first to define at least some borderline subgroups that did not bear some direct or even indirect relationship to schizophrenia.

The term borderline, nonetheless, did not become well known until Kernberg developed his theory of borderline personality organization (Kernberg 1967). It is of interest that although Kernberg's theory of borderline personality organization (BPO) popularized the word as well as the concept of "borderline," Kernberg was not describing a diagnostic entity. Rather, BPO, strongly rooted in object relations theory, was an overarching concept that could encompass a wide variety of patients with character pathology, and BPO was not specific to those patients who would meet the current DSM-III or DSM-III-R (American Psychiatric Association 1987) diagnosis of BPD.

However, it was not until the mid-1970s that a series of empirical studies, conducted primarily by Gunderson (Gunderson and Singer 1975; Gunderson and Kolb 1978) and Perry and Klerman (1978, 1980), defined and operationalized a set of criteria that would lead to a formalized and accepted diagnosis of BPD. Researchers cannot study a disorder until it is defined, and yet, in the case of BPD, psychiatric clinicians and investigators needed to finally settle on a working definition of the disorder in order to study it. This process of agreeing on some formal definition of BPD has been completed, as indicated by the criteria set in DSM-III, but the diagnosis also continues to evolve, since diagnosis in psychiatry is a process of constant refinement.

The discussion surrounding diagnosis of the personality disorders has been an interesting one. The argument has been made that personality disorders—especially BPD—are atypical manifestations of Axis I disorders, and that there is no or little need for a separate axis, let alone a separate set of diagnoses (Akiskal et al. 1985a). However, the fact that there was an official set of personality disorder diagnostic categories in DSM-III has led to a series of refinements in classification of personality disorders that will be particularly noticeable in DSM-IV (American Psychiatric Association 1994). Clinicians and researchers acknowledge that our diagnostic categories always prove to be limited when challenged by the wide variety of ways in which patients present themselves to us. Although we define our patients in categories that we hope are reflective of the actual "genotype," our patients often do not present with symptomatology that falls into distinct diagnostic categories. Phenotypic or clinical presentation by our patients often appears more dimensional than categorical (Gunderson et al. 1991). Patients repeatedly fail to read the DSM before presenting themselves to us in clinical practice.

This empirical work of the 1970s led to a more narrow definition of BPD as compared with Kernberg's BPO. Attempts were made to separate out this more narrow definition of BPD from the "borderline" diagnoses of the past, which seemed more closely related to schizophrenia. The borderline diagnosis became "official" with the publication of DSM-III, in which the "borderline" label was reserved for the more interpersonally unstable, affectively labile patients (Spitzer et al. 1979). Patients more closely connected to schizophrenia—and probably more closely related to the descriptions of borderline patients prior to the mid-1960s—were classified under *schizotypal personality disorder*. This separation of borderline patients into schizotypal and affectively unstable subtypes was not without its problems, and there remains a substantial group of patients (as high as 50%) who meet the criteria for both diagnostic categories (Kavoussi and Siever 1992; Silk et al. 1990). It is hoped that the revised criteria in DSM-IV for both schizotypal and borderline (unstable) personality disorder will reduce some of this diagnostic overlap.

Nonetheless, the work of Gunderson and Singer and of Spitzer et al. allowed a clearer definition of what constituted BPD and led to the development of the Diagnostic Interview for Borderlines (DIB; Gunderson et al. 1981) and a number of other operationalized instruments for diagnosing BPD (Reich 1989). The DIB and its successor, the DIB-R (Zanarini et al. 1989b), currently the most frequently utilized structured instruments for the diagnosis of BPD, have excellent interrater and test–retest reliability (Cornell et al. 1983; Zanarini et al. 1989b). Eighty percent of patients diagnosed as borderline by the DIB also meet the DSM-III-R criteria for BPD.

The development of a reliable diagnostic instrument allowed clinicians and researchers to isolate a group of patients for further study, and one of the key areas for exploration was research into the biological processes that may be occurring in borderline patients. Patients diagnosed as borderline by either the DSM or the DIB were more affective-appearing (Stone 1979), even if affectively unstable. The initial studies that sought to understand biological processes in BPD began by applying to borderline patients those biological probes that were being studied in affective patients at that time.

The first areas of biological inquiry into BPD involved the dexamethasone suppression test (DST), the response of thyrotropin-stimulating hormone to thyrotropin-releasing hormone (the TRH test), and the study of early onset rapid eye movement (REM) latency periods in the sleep electroencephalograms (EEGs) of borderline patients. Although the DST has been shown to be positive across all studies in 20%–80% of borderline patients (Baxter et al. 1984; Carroll et al. 1981; Silk et al. 1985; Soloff et al. 1982; Sternbach et al. 1983; Val et al. 1983), in prospective studies using structured interviews for the diagnosis of BPD, only 24% of borderline patients, on average, have positive DSTs (Silk et al. 1985). Some studies found that a positive DST closely followed the comorbid diagnosis of affective disorder in these patients (Baxter et al. 1984; Krishnan et al. 1984), whereas in other studies the co-occurrence of a positive DST and a comorbid diagnosis of mood disorder was a much rarer finding (Beeber et al. 1984; Nathan et al. 1986; Silk et al. 1985; Soloff et al. 1982). A similar lack of concordance between a test thought to be positive in affective disorder and a comorbid diagnosis of affective disorder in borderline patients occurred in the two studies of the TRH test in borderline patients (Garbutt et al. 1983; Sternbach et al. 1983).

However, the results of sleep studies exploring REM latency show a closer, but not entirely clearer, link between borderline and affective patients. There has been, to my knowledge, only one study that did not find shortened REM latency among patients with BPD, regardless of the comorbid diagnosis of affective disorder, although in that study (Benson et al. 1990), borderline patients who also met criteria for major depression had an REM latency of 54.8 minutes compared with that of the nondepressed borderline patients and of the nonpsychiatrically ill control subjects (76 minutes and 94 minutes, respectively). Six other studies (Akiskal et al. 1985b; Bell et al. 1983; Lahmeyer et al. 1988; McNamara et al. 1984; Reynolds et al. 1985; Silk et al. 1988) found no significant difference between the REM latencies of borderline patients and those of depressed patients, although again the results are confounded by the issue of affective comorbidity among the borderline subjects. While many of these studies attempted to separate out depressed from nondepressed borderline patients (Akiskal et al. 1985b; Reynolds et al. 1985), it was very difficult to demarcate a group of borderline patients who did not have chronic dysthymia or who had no affective episodes in the past (Akiskal et al. 1985b; Perry 1985; Zanarini et al. 1989a), perhaps because both the DSM-III and the DIB criteria heavily depend on affective symptoms or perhaps because of a true biological relationship between the two disorders. Yet despite the fact that a similar shortening of REM latencies occurred in both the borderline and the depressed groups, the sleep abnormality results among the borderline patients were independent of the level of depressive symptomatology (Akiskal et al. 1985b; Reynolds et al. 1985; Silk et al. 1988), a situation not found among "pure" depressed patients, in whom REM latencies are inversely correlated with Hamilton Rating Scale for Depression (HRSD; Hamilton 1960) scores (Reynolds et al. 1985).

Whereas attention was focused by some on the biological, neuroendocrinological, or electrophysiological relationship between affective disorder patients and borderline patients, others were exploring how borderline patients responded to the "standard" pharmacological treatments for depression. Again, however, in this arena as well, patients with BPD in some respects looked like depressed patients but did not appear to respond to antidepressant medications as "pure" depressed patients responded. Soloff et al. (1986b) found that not only was amitriptyline not as effective as a low-dose neuroleptic in the treatment of borderline depressed patients, but some of these patients appeared to get worse on a tricyclic antidepressant (Soloff et al. 1986a). The beneficial effect of low-dose neuroleptics has been shown in a number of studies (Goldberg et al. 1986; Serban and Siegal 1984; Soloff et al. 1986b). Further, although many of the symptoms alleviated by the low-dose neuroleptics related to hostility and impulsivity, there was also a significant improvement in depressive symptomatology (Soloff et al. 1986b). In fact, Soloff's initial studies supported the idea that low-dose neuroleptics were significantly more effective than placebo across all symptom domains. More recently, this group of researchers has concluded that haloperidol works best in the most severely symptomatic borderline patients. Low-dose neuroleptics may be less effective in less severely disturbed borderline patients and less effective than originally thought against depressive symptomatology (Soloff 1993; Soloff et al. 1993), although, in my clinical experience, patients taking low-dose neuroleptics often report being able to "focus better" cognitively on a given intellectual task or to better concentrate and therefore better comprehend what other people say.

Thus, the initial biological approaches centered on the relationship of BPD to the mood disorders. However, the results both of the biological and of the pharmacological studies revealed that borderline patients were at best extremely "atypical" in their biological correspondence to depressed patients.

This book presents what I would like to call the "second generation" of biological and neurobehavioral studies of borderline patients. Rather than focusing on the borderline patient's relationship to a specific diagnostic category, these more recent studies explore the purported biological underpinnings of dimensions of psychopathology frequently found in characterologically disturbed patients.

Van Reekum and colleagues explore the centrality and reliability of the term *impulsivity* in relation to borderline criteria and suggest that the classic impulsivity seen among borderline patients has much in common with impulsivity as displayed in some organic brain disorders. DeVegvar et al. report on studies of the biological underpinnings of impulsivity and aggression, particularly as they relate to disturbances in serotonin regulation. Steinberg and colleagues, from the same research group as deVegvar, present recent evidence supporting a relationship between cholinergic hypersensitivity and affective lability; they also report research findings that implicate noradrenergic mechanisms in affective lability. Yehuda et al. present data supporting alterations in peripheral catecholamine activity in BPD and propose that these alterations support a relationship of BPD to posttraumatic stress disorder (PTSD) and perhaps to other anxiety disorders as well. Silk and colleagues discuss the relationship between BPD and anxiety and panic disorders and present preliminary data on lactate-induced panic attacks in criteria-defined borderline subjects. Goyer et al. review the early but developing state of neuroimaging in borderline and other personality disorders and speculate on how, in the future, these neuroimaging techniques may help us to better "localize" those areas of the brain most suspect in initiation or maintenance of some borderline psychopathology. O'Leary and Cowdry compare and discuss four studies that explore neuropsychological test performance among borderline patients. Zanarini and colleagues explore, through chart review, neurological dysfunction among borderline patients. Teicher et al. report evidence of limbic system dysfunction among borderline patients with a history of childhood abuse; the authors present an intriguing hypothesis concerning the relationship of abuse to limbic system dysfunction and its clinical manifestations as borderline symptomatology. Cowdry reviews all of these studies and reflects on the future course of biological and neurobehavioral research in BPD.

Finally, as a sort of epilogue, Silk discusses how the studies in this volume might impact upon our clinical evaluation and care of borderline patients and how they might inform our pharmacological choices as well.

It is hoped that this volume will have current as well as historical value. From a current perspective, it presents and reviews the most recent inquiries into the biological and neurological underpinnings of dimensions of psychopathology found among borderline patients. Because the neurobiological study of these dimensions is only beginning, this book represents a historical collection of early biological explorations into the nature of borderline and other personality disorders. Perhaps in the not-too-distant future these studies will seem crude or simplistic. Nonetheless, they may serve as the jumping-off place for future research into the biology of personality disorders.

References

Akiskal HS: Subaffective disorders: dysthymic, cyclothymic, and bipolar II disorders in the "borderline" realm. Psychiatr Clin North Am 4:25–46, 1981

Akiskal HS, Chen SE, David GC, et al: Borderline: an adjective in search of a noun. J Clin Psychiatry 46:41–48, 1985a

Akiskal HS, Yerevanian BI, Davis GC: The nosologic status of borderline personality: clinical and polysomnographic study. Am J Psychiatry 142:192–198, 1985b

American Psychiatric Association: Diagnostic and Statistical Manual of Mental Disorders, 3rd Edition. Washington, DC, American Psychiatric Association, 1980

American Psychiatric Association: Diagnostic and Statistical Manual of Mental Disorders, 3rd Edition, Revised. Washington, DC, American Psychiatric Association, 1987

American Psychiatric Association: Diagnostic and Statistical Manual of Mental Disorders, 4th Edition. Washington, DC, American Psychiatric Association, 1994

Baxter L, Edell W, Gerner R, et al: Dexamethasone suppression test and Axis I diagnoses of inpatients with DSM-III borderline personality disorder. J Clin Psychiatry 45:150–153, 1984

Beeber AR, Kline MD, Pies RW, et al: Dexamethasone suppression test in hospitalized depressed patients with borderline personality disorder. J Nerv Ment Dis 172:301–303, 1984

Bell J, Lycaki H, Jones D, et al: Effect of preexisting borderline personality disorder on clinical and EEG sleep correlates of depression. Psychiatry Res 9:115–123, 1983

Benson KL, King R, Gordon D, et al: Sleep patterns in borderline personality disorder. J Affective Disord 18:267–273, 1990

Carroll BJ, Greden JF, Feinberg M, et al: Neuroendocrine evaluation of depression in borderline patients. Psychiatr Clin North Am 4:89–99, 1981

Cornell DG, Silk KR, Ludolph PS, et al: Test–retest reliability of the diagnostic interview for borderlines. Arch Gen Psychiatry 40:1307–1310, 1983

Cowdry RW, Gardner DL: Pharmacotherapy of borderline personality disorder: alprazolam, carbamazepine, trifluoperazine and tranylcypromine. Arch Gen Psychiatry 45:111–119, 1988

Deutsch H: Some forms of emotional disturbance and their relationship to schizophrenia. Psychoanal Q 11:301–321, 1942

Dulit RA, Fyer MR, Haas GL, et al: Substance use in borderline personality disorder. Am J Psychiatry 147:1002–1007, 1990

Garbutt JC, Loosen PT, Tipermas A, et al: The TRH test in patients with borderline personality disorder. Psychiatry Res 9:107–113, 1983

Goldberg SC, Schulz SC, Schulz PM, et al: Borderline and schizotypal personality disorders treated with low-dose thiothixene vs placebo. Arch Gen Psychiatry 43:680–686, 1986

Grinker RR, Werble B, Drye RC: The Borderline Syndrome: A Behavioral Study of Ego Functions. New York, Basic Books, 1968

Gunderson JG: Pharmacotherapy for patients with borderline personality disorder. Arch Gen Psychiatry 43:698–700, 1986

Gunderson JG, Elliott GR: The interface between borderline personality disorder and affective disorder. Am J Psychiatry 142:277–288, 1985

Gunderson JG, Kolb JE: Discriminating features of borderline patients. Am J Psychiatry 135:792–796, 1978

Gunderson JG, Singer MT: Defining borderline patients: an overview. Am J Psychiatry 132:1–10, 1975

Gunderson JG, Kolb JE, Austin V: The Diagnostic Interview for Borderline Patients. Am J Psychiatry 138:896–903, 1981

Gunderson JG, Links PS, Reich JH: Competing models of personality disorders. Journal of Personality Disorders 5:60–68, 1991

Hamilton M: A rating scale for depression. J Neurol Neurosurg Psychiatry 23:56–62, 1960

Hoch P, Polatin P: Pseudoneurotic forms of schizophrenia. Psychiatr Q 23:248–276, 1949

Kavoussi RJ, Siever LJ: Overlap between borderline and schizotypal personality disorders. Compr Psychiatry 33:7–12, 1992

Kernberg OF: Borderline personality organization. J Am Psychoanal Assoc 15:641–685, 1967

Kernberg O: Borderline Conditions and Pathological Narcissism. New York, Jason Aronson, 1975

Knight R: Borderline states. Bull Menninger Clin 17:1–12, 1953

Krishnan KR, Davidson JRT, Rayasam K, et al: The dexamethasone suppression test in borderline personality disorder. Biol Psychiatry 19:1149–1153, 1984

Lahmeyer HW, Val E, Gaviria M, et al: EEG sleep, lithium transport, dexamethasone suppression and monoamine oxidase activity in borderline personality disorder. Psychiatry Res 25:19–30, 1988

McNamara E, Reynolds CF III, Soloff PH, et al: EEG sleep evaluation of depression in borderline patients. Am J Psychiatry 141:182–186, 1984

Main TF: The ailment. Br J Med Psychol 30:129–145, 1957

Nathan RS, Soloff PH, George A, et al: DST and TRH tests in borderline personality disorder, in Biological Psychiatry: Proceedings of the 4th World Congress of Biological Psychiatry. Edited by Shagass C, Josiassen RG, Wagner BH, et al. New York, Elsevier, 1986, pp 564–565

Perry JC: Depression in borderline personality disorder: lifetime prevalence at interview and longitudinal course of symptoms. Am J Psychiatry 142:15–21, 1985

Perry JC, Klerman GL: The borderline patient. Arch Gen Psychiatry 35:141–150, 1978

Perry JC, Klerman GL: Clinical features of the borderline personality disorder. Am J Psychiatry 137:165–173, 1980

Reich J: Update on instruments to measure DSM-III and DSM-III-R personality disorders. J Nerv Ment Dis 177:366–371, 1989

Reynolds CF III, Soloff PH, Kupfer DJ, et al: Depression in borderline patients: a prospective EEG sleep study. Psychiatry Res 14:1–15, 1985

Serban G, Siegel S: Response of borderline and schizotypal patients to small doses of thiothixene and haloperidol. Am J Psychiatry 141:1455–1458, 1984

Silk KR, Lohr NE, Cornell DG, et al: The dexamethasone suppression test in borderline and nonborderline affective patients, in The Borderline: Current Empirical Research. Edited by McGlashan T. Washington, DC, American Psychiatric Press, 1985, pp 99–116

Silk KR, Lohr NE, Shipley JE, et al: Sleep EEG and DST in borderlines with depression. Paper presented at the 141st annual meeting of the American Psychiatric Association, Montreal, Canada, May 1988

Silk KR, Cohen R, Gold L, et al: Psychotic symptoms in borderline personality disorder: consideration for DSM-IV (abstract). Biol Psychiatry 25 (no 7A):88A, 1989

Silk KR, Westen D, Lohr NE, et al: DSM-III and DSM-III-R schizotypal symptoms in borderline personality disorder. Compr Psychiatry 31:103–110, 1990

Soloff PH: Pharmacological therapies in borderline personality disorder, in Borderline Personality Disorder: Etiology and Treatment. Edited by Paris J. Washington, DC, American Psychiatric Press, 1993, pp 319–348

Soloff PH, George A, Nathan R: Dexamethasone suppression test in patients with borderline personality disorder. Am J Psychiatry 139:1621–1622, 1982

Soloff PH, George A, Nathan R, et al: Paradoxical effects of amitriptyline in borderline patients. Am J Psychiatry 143:1603–1605, 1986a

Soloff PH, George A, Nathan R, et al: Progress in the pharmacotherapy of borderline disorders. Arch Gen Psychiatry 43:691–697, 1986b

Soloff PH, Cornelius J, George A, et al: Efficacy of phenelzine and haloperidol in borderline personality disorder. Arch Gen Psychiatry 50:377–385, 1993

Spitzer RL, Endicott J, Gibbon M: Crossing the border into borderline personality and borderline schizophrenia: the development of criteria. Arch Gen Psychiatry 36:17–24, 1979

Stern A: Psychoanalytic investigation of and therapy in the borderline group of neuroses. Psychoanal Q 7:467–489, 1938

Sternbach HA, Fleming J, Extein I, et al: The dexamethasone suppression and thyrotropin-releasing hormone tests in depressed borderline patients. Psychoneuroendocrinology 8:459–462, 1983

Stone MH: Contemporary shift of the borderline concept from a subschizophrenic disorder to a subaffective disorder. Psychiatr Clin North Am 2:577–594, 1979

Val ER, Nasr SJ, Gaviria FW, et al: Depression, borderline disorder, and the DST (letter). Am J Psychiatry 140:819, 1983

Zanarini MC: BPD as an impulse spectrum disorder, in Borderline Personality Disorder: Etiology and Treatment. Edited by Paris J. Washington, DC, American Psychiatric Press, 1993, pp 67–85

Zanarini MC, Gunderson JG, Frankenburg FR: Axis I phenomenology of borderline personality disorder. Compr Psychiatry 30:149–156, 1989a

Zanarini MC, Gunderson JG, Frankenburg FR, et al: The revised diagnostic interview for borderlines: discriminating BPD from other Axis II disorders. Journal of Personality Disorders 3:10–18, 1989b

Zanarini MC, Gunderson JG, Frankenberg FR: Cognitive features of borderline personality disorder. Am J Psychiatry 147:57–63, 1990

Zilboorg G: Ambulatory schizophrenia. Psychiatry 4:149–155, 1941

Chapter 1

Impulsivity in Borderline Personality Disorder

Robert van Reekum, M.D., F.R.C.P.C.
Paul S. Links, M.D., F.R.C.P.C.
Cecilia Fedorov, R.N.

Impulsivity and its related concepts (e.g., aggression) have long been recognized as core diagnostic features of borderline personality disorder (BPD) (American Psychiatric Association 1980; Gunderson et al. 1981; Kernberg 1975, 1976). More recently, the suggestion has been made that impulsivity may be central to the pathogenesis of BPD (Gunderson and Phillips 1991; Gunderson and Zanarini 1989; Links and Boiago 1990). Family history studies (reviewed by Gunderson and Zanarini 1989; Links and Boiago 1990), studies of cognitive functioning in BPD (Burgess 1991), and biological marker studies (Coccaro et al. 1989; Gardner et al. 1990) have begun to elucidate the biological underpinnings of impulsivity in BPD.

These studies are promising in that a greater understanding of the pathogenesis and etiology of impulsivity in BPD may lead to the development of new treatment modalities for this common and difficult-to-treat disorder. For example, Cowdry and Gardner (1988) have demonstrated a decrease in behavioral dyscontrol with carbamazepine in BPD. Three open trials with fluoxetine showed improvement in impulsivity in BPD (Cornelius et al. 1990; Markovitz et al. 1991; Norden 1989). Impulsivity also improved during a preliminary randomized clinical trial with lithium (Links et al. 1990a). Linehan's dialectical behavior therapy (DBT; Linehan et al. 1991) shows promise of being able to reduce the frequency and severity of parasuicides. These early and preliminary studies of possible treatments of impulsivity in BPD support the need for further research into both the causes of and the treatments for this core feature of BPD.

These endeavors are hampered at present by a lack of consensus as to the exact nature of impulsivity in BPD and by a lack of understanding regarding the relationship of impulsivity to outcome in BPD. Clinicians should be committed to treating not only those symptoms/behaviors that are problematic in the here and now but also those symptoms/behaviors that have been shown to have or that may have a relationship with the outcome of the disorder.

In this chapter we address questions as to the nature of impulsivity in BPD and the relationship of impulsivity to outcome, first through a review of the relevant literature, and then by a secondary analysis of data derived from a 5-year prospective follow-up study of BPD. This prospective follow-up study is currently in progress at McMaster University (Hamilton, Ontario) under the directorship of Dr. Paul Links. Outcome, in this case, will be defined as current social functioning as well as current (cross-sectional) diagnosis of BPD.

THE NATURE OF IMPULSIVITY IN BPD

Although the term *impulsivity* is widely used, it lacks diagnostic specificity. Health care workers, including pediatricians and other child-care providers, psychologists, psychiatrists, and neurologists, are frequently confronted by disordered behavior or cognition to which is attached the label of impulsivity. Different conceptual bases among—and even within—these fields lead naturally to a lack of precision in using the term. Use of the term appears to span the range from the rapid, poorly planned response style revealed in test taking and noted by neuropsychologists, through disinhibited affects such as irritability and affective lability, to more overt behaviors such as reckless driving and other thrill-seeking behaviors, and, finally, culminating in behavior central to diagnosis—that is, at the level of syndrome or disorder, as found in substance use disorders, antisocial personality disorder, and orbital frontal syndrome.

In DSM-III (American Psychiatric Association 1980) and DSM-III-R (American Psychiatric Association 1987), impulsivity is a principal diagnostic feature in many categories of disorders: childhood disorders (attention-deficit hyperactivity disorder [ADHD]), organic mental disorders, disorders of impulse control not otherwise specified, and personality disorders (borderline or antisocial or histrionic personality disorder). Further, impulsivity is frequently associated with many other disorders such as "agitated" depression, psychoses, psychosexual disorders, and so forth. The diagnostic nonspecificity of such a broad concept is inevitable.

Application of the term *impulsivity* to a specific disorder such as BPD has been complicated by a lack of agreement as to how to measure impulsivity. Various measures have been used. The Diagnostic Interview for Borderlines (DIB; Gunderson et al. 1981), and its revised version, the DIB-R (Zanarini et al. 1989), are widely accepted diagnostic instruments for BPD. In the DIB and DIB-R, impulsivity is measured primarily in the impulse action subscale, although the theme of impulsivity is noted in other subscales, such as in the affect subscale under affective lability and irritability. Within the impulse action subscale, impulsivity is measured by evidence of substance abuse, sexual deviance, self-mutilation, manipulative suicidal efforts or threats, and a "catchall" category that includes accident proneness, eating binges, spending/gambling sprees, poor temper control, fights, threats/assaults, reckless driving, and antisocial behavior.

The Structured Interview for DSM-III-R Personality Disorders (SIDP-R; Pfohl et al. 1989) is a widely used instrument designed to assess DSM-III-R personality disorders. As with the DSM-III-R, on the SIDP-R patients require the presence of five of eight criteria to meet the diagnosis of BPD. The theme of impulsivity appears in five of the eight items: unstable and intense interpersonal relationships; affective instability; inappropriate and/or intense anger or lack of control of anger; recurrent suicidal threats, gestures, or behavior, or self-mutilating behavior; and impulsiveness in at least two of the following areas: childhood conduct problems, spending, sex, substance use, antisocial behavior, binge eating, irritability, aggression, poor planning, irresponsible parenting, relationship instability, and work instability. Clearly, the DIB/DIB-R and the DSM-III-R, as measured by the SIDP-R, are assessing a very wide range of behaviors and affects in order to determine the presence of impulsivity. Patients meeting the impulsivity criteria may be exhibiting any of a number of these behaviors, and thus comparisons between patients and between groups of BPD patients are complicated and confounded.

Researchers interested in the phenomenon of impulsivity in BPD have employed other measures of impulsivity in an attempt to narrow the scope of the concept and to make connections to specific elements within the global concept of impulsivity. Gardner and colleagues (1991) used the Buss-Durkee Hostility Inventory (BDHI; Buss and Durkee 1957) to demonstrate that BPD patients from a variety of clinical settings are more irritable and show more negativism, resentment, suspicion, and guilt than do nonpsychiatrically ill control subjects. Borderline patients did not differ from control subjects on the assault, indirect hostility, and verbal hostility subscales. BPD patients' scores were not related to gender, treatment setting, degree of acute distress, or the presence of comorbid major depression.

Buss and Durkee (1957) recognized a lack of precision in the use of the term *hostility* (which they also used interchangeably with the term *aggression*). The BDHI measures hostility in eight subscales derived from 75 items. Factor analysis revealed two factors: 1) an "emotion" or attitudinal factor composed of the resentment and suspicion (and, in women, the guilt) subscales, and 2) a "motor" factor composed of the assault, indirect hostility, irritability, and verbal hostility (and, in women, the negativism) subscales. The average factor loadings, however, were not high in these studies, which were derived from a sample of college students.

Gardner et al.'s (1991) results reveal that BPD subjects differ from control subjects in all three subscales that make up the attitudinal, or emotion, factor of hostility. While the BPD subjects also differed on the irritability and negativism subscales of the motor factor, a careful review of the individual items comprised in these two subscales suggests that these are the least "motoric" of the subscales included in the motor factor. Gardner et al.'s results thus suggest that "anger" is central to the concept of impulsivity in BPD, and that anger is a stable feature that is independent of depressive affective state in BPD. Limitations of this study include the fact that two of the three cohorts of borderline patients specifically excluded physically assaultive patients, and one of these two cohorts was specifically chosen by incorporating into the inclusion criteria the presence of self-injurious and impulsive dyscontrol. In this study, the BDHI was used as a self-report measure, and such use of the measure raises the possibility of social desirability biases. However, the conclusions of the study are supported by other studies that have examined anger in BPD (Gunderson et al. 1975; Perry and Klerman 1980) and by previous research that used the BDHI with borderline patients (Soloff 1981a, 1981b).

Efforts to associate particular elements of impulsivity in BPD with factors other than the diagnosis of BPD have focused primarily on the relationship of impulsivity to neurotransmitter functioning and pharmacological response. Coccaro et al. (1989) showed significant negative correlations between peak changes in prolactin responses to fenfluramine (a measure of central nervous system [CNS] serotonergic activity) and BDHI motor aggression, lifetime aggression as measured by the Brown-Goodwin Assessment for Life History of Aggression (BGA; Brown et al. 1979), and "impulsiveness" as measured by the Barratt Impulsivity Scale (BIS; Barratt 1965). The BIS, now in its 10th revision (Barratt 1990), is a 34-item self-report instrument from which are derived three subscales: motor, cognitive, and nonplanning. The motor subscale taps behaviors that reveal themselves as acting without thinking; the cognitive subscale evaluates processes such as making up one's mind too quickly; and the nonplanning subscale probes attitudes such as living for the moment without planning ahead. In Coccaro et al.'s (1989) study, analysis of individual BDHI and BIS subscale contributions to the inverse correlations with prolactin revealed that the BDHI assault and irritability subscales and the BIS motor impulsiveness subscale accounted for most of the variance seen in prolactin response. These three subscales, furthermore, were highly correlated with the BGA score. These intercorrelations among certain subscales of the BDHI, the BIS, and the BGA suggest that these measures are assessing strongly related phenomena (Coccaro et al. 1991).

Gardner et al. (1990) showed a relationship between low cerebrospinal fluid (CSF) levels of 5-hydroxyindoleacetic acid (5-HIAA), a serotonin metabolite, and a history of genuine suicide attempts. No correlations were found with other CSF metabolites or with other elements of impulsivity such as violence and self-mutilation. These elements of impulsivity were measured by nonstructured clinical interview. Comparing these results with the results from Coccaro's group is complicated because different measures/concepts of impulsivity were used and different measures were employed to assess serotonergic functioning.

In a closely related field of study, Burgess (1991) showed an association between self-injury in BPD and poorer performance on cognitive tests of attention and memory. Self-injury was evaluated with an 11-item scale that measured the presence or absence of a range of self-injurious behaviors. It will be interesting to extend this area of research to include studies of possible relationships between cognitive and neurotransmitter functioning in "impulsive" BPD patients.

Cowdry and Gardner (1988), in a double-blind crossover study of 16 women with BPD who had a history of "extensive behavioral dyscontrol," used physician ratings on a seven-point scale to evaluate degree of improvement in "impulsivity" among patients treated with carbamazepine or tranylcypromine (as well as with other pharmacological agents). Improvement on a seven-point "suicidality" scale was demonstrated in patients treated with these two medications as well as in patients treated with trifluoperazine. The authors also tried to rate the severity of the worst episode of "actual behavioral dyscontrol" during each medication trial; behaviors measured included angry outbursts, physical violence, self-damaging acts, and suicidal gestures. Only those patients taking carbamazepine showed a "dramatic," highly statistically significant improvement in the severity of actual behavioral dyscontrol.

Cornelius and his colleagues (1990) failed to find any improvement in hostility as measured by the BDHI among five BPD patients treated with fluoxetine in an open trial. However, hostility as measured by the hospital subscale of the Hopkins Symptom Checklist—90 (SCL-90; Derogatis et al. 1973) did show improvement. "State impulsiveness" as recorded by the Ward Scale of Impulse Action Patterns, a measure developed by Soloff and his colleagues (1986), also improved. The Ward Scale is based on the impulse action subscale of the DIB (Gunderson et al. 1981) and lists 12 behavioral symptoms (e.g., assaultiveness, manipulativeness, self-mutilation, temper tantrums, suicide threats) frequently displayed by patients with BPD during their hospital stays (Soloff et al. 1986). This scale had been used by Soloff et al. (1986, 1987) to measure a decrease in impulsivity among BPD inpatients treated with low-dose haloperidol.

This brief review of the relationship of impulsivity, particularly in BPD, to neurotransmitters, cognitive functioning, and pharmacological response serves to illustrate the methodological difficulties inherent in employing such a broad, poorly defined concept of impulsivity. It is almost impossible to compare studies that use differing measures as well as different concepts of impulsivity. More preliminary work to define the nature of impulsivity in BPD, such as the research done by Gardner et al. (1991), is needed. For example, Coccaro et al.'s (1989) work with serotonin suggests that serotonergic system manipulation may improve impulsivity in BPD. However, the type of impulsivity most strongly associated with low serotonergic activity—motoric aggression—was not found by Gardner et al. (1991) to be more common in BPD patients than in control subjects (although the Gardner et al. study did show selection bias as noted above). Irritability, as measured by the BDHI, was nevertheless more common in BPD patients than in control subjects (Gardner et al. 1991), and this facet of impulsivity is associated with low serotonergic activity (Coccaro et al. 1989). Among borderline patients, then, irritability may be both more common and more amenable to treatment with serotonergic agents than among patients without a personality disorder.

When we consider treatment of impulsivity or other symptoms of BPD, we should try to direct our treatment not only to those impulsive behaviors that are found to be common in BPD, but also to those behaviors that have been found to be associated with poor outcome. In the next section we look at the relationship of impulsivity to outcome in borderline patients.

THE RELATIONSHIP OF IMPULSIVITY TO OUTCOME IN BPD

The relationship of impulsivity and other prognostic variables to outcome in borderline personality disorder has been reviewed elsewhere (Stone 1989). In this section we highlight some of Stone's findings as well as examine results from research not reviewed by Stone (Links et al. 1990b).

Among borderline patients, substance abuse appears to increase the suicide rate and to decrease the chances of recovery (Stone et al. 1988). The presence of comorbid antisocial personality is likewise "associated with a dismal prognosis" (Stone 1989, p. 115). Severity of impulsivity and self-damaging behavior at index evaluation also predicts successful suicide (Stone et al. 1988), as does a history of repeated suicide attempts (Kotila and Lonnquist 1987). Borderline patients with a history of fire setting (an antisocial criterion) during childhood have a poorer long-term outcome than BPD patients who lack this childhood behavior.

Links et al. (1990b) performed a 2-year follow-up study of BPD. This study included the use of a prospective design to ensure systematic time 1 data collection, a broad range of sample sources, and structured outcome assessments. Patients were referred from a variety of inpatient settings in Hamilton, Ontario. Of the original 130 patients recruited, 88 were DIB-positive for a diagnosis of borderline personality disorder at time 1. Sixty-five (74% of the 88) patients were followed up a mean of 20.6 months later. The outcome measures used included the DIB and McGlashan's Total Follow-Up Period Outcome Dimensions (McGlashan 1984). The McGlashan scale assesses five aspects of outcome: time spent in hospital or halfway home, employment, social activity, psychopathology, and overall global functioning.

Four of the study's probands committed suicide. Poor outcome was defined as functioning normally less than 50% of the follow-up period based on the overall global assessment of McGlashan. Dropouts ($n = 19$) were differentiated from the follow-up group on several variables, including the presence of a comorbid diagnosis of antisocial personality disorder. Nevertheless, in the sample followed, the poor-outcome probands had histories of significantly more antisocial behaviors before 15 years of age. In addition, when compared with the good-outcome probands, those with poor outcomes had higher impulse action scores based on initial DIB assessment and were found, at index, to have poorer premorbid functioning (as manifested by occupational status, school performance, marital status, and absences from work). Other postulated predictor variables—history of abuse, disrupted family environment, gender, IQ, previous psychiatric history, substance abuse, major depression, and labile personality—did not predict poor outcome. Furthermore, when the categories of alcoholism, drug use, and antisocial and borderline personality disorders were assessed (taken together as a group) in the first-degree relatives of the probands, the frequency of these diagnoses was also related to poor outcome in the probands (odds ratio = 3.25, 95% confidence interval = 1.16–9.09). These four variables—significant antisocial behaviors before the age of 15, high index DIB impulse action subscale scores, poor premorbid functioning, and familial "impulsive" diagnoses—were entered into a logistic regression model to predict poor versus good outcome. Two variables—high impulse action scores and poor premorbid functioning—remained in the model at $P < .10$.

Thus, both the outcome study by Stone (1989) and the outcome study done here in Hamilton, Ontario (Links et al. [1990b]) suggest a prognostic role for some elements of impulsivity in BPD. However, our review has focused only on impulsivity as a predictor of outcome, and other significant predictive variables exist. In addition, not all outcome studies have shown that impulsivity has a predictive role (McGlashan 1985; Paris et at. 1987). Nonetheless, substance abuse, comorbid antisocial personality disorder, a history of childhood conduct problems, high index impulse action scores on the DIB, recurrent suicide attempts, and a family history of impulse disorders have all been shown to be possible predictors of poor outcome in BPD. It should be noted that in these studies as well as those discussed in the previous sections, the definition of impulsivity was not consistent across studies, and the interrelationships of these clinical manifestations of impulsivity in BPD are not yet understood.

THE CURRENT STUDY

Objectives and Analyses

The study presented in this section was an exploratory study and had no *a priori* hypotheses. We undertook the study with the hope of answering two groups of questions:

1. Which of several measures of impulsivity best correlates (Pearson correlations) with the DIB impulse action subscale score in a cohort of BPD subjects? Furthermore, how well do these non-DIB measures of impulsivity correlate with the total DIB score? Answers to these questions will contribute to our understanding of a) the nature of impulsivity in BPD, b) the behavioral characteristics of BPD patients who score positively on the DIB impulse action subscale, and c) the relationship of the overall DIB symptom complex to impulsivity.
2. Which of several measures of impulsivity best predicts current functioning, and what contribution does impulsivity make to functioning? Functioning will be defined as ongoing BPD characteristics as measured both by the DIB and by measures of social functioning. Answers to these questions will help to determine the contribution of various aspects of impulsivity to the BPD diagnosis and to social functioning, and the results may focus research and clinical efforts on those elements of impulsivity in BPD that bear a relationship to current functioning. Data will be analyzed by stepwise multiple regression with limits to enter the model set at $P < .05$.

Subjects

Subjects were derived from a 5-year prospective follow-up study of BPD currently in progress that represents a continuation of the 2-year follow-up study discussed previously. Subjects and initial methodology have been presented in previous publications (Links et al. 1990b). Briefly, the initial cohort was referred from any of four inpatient psychiatric facilities associated with McMaster University, Faculty of Health Sciences, Department of

Psychiatry, Hamilton, Ontario. Referral was based on a suspected diagnosis of BPD. Of 130 referred subjects, 88 scored 7 on the DIB (Gunderson et al. 1981). These 88 probands were reassessed at 2 years (Links et al. 1990b), and all 126 survivors were asked to participate in further follow-up 5–7 years postindex contact. An informative letter was followed by telephone requests to participate. Data are now available on 57 of the BPD cohort. Most interviews were done in person ($n = 47$); 10 were done by telephone.

Methods

All subjects signed an informed consent. The clinical research nurse conducting the interviews was blind to all diagnoses and histories obtained during both the initial and the first follow-up period (2 years). Interview-based outcome (functioning) measures included the following:

1. The Global Assessment Scale (GAS; Endicott et al. 1976) was used to rate each subject's overall functioning, from 1 to 100, for the week before the interview.
2. The DIB (Gunderson et al. 1981) was used for the initial diagnosis of BPD and again at 2 years and at this 5-year follow-up. At the time of this current phase of the study, the revised DIB—the DIB-R (Zanarini et al. 1989)—had become available. We opted to use a combination of the DIB and the DIB-R (items that were the same in both instruments were used only once).
3. The Suicidal Behaviors Questionnaire (SBQ; Linehan 1983), an interview-based predictive measure, was used to assess each subject's self-harm/suicidal ideation in the previous 6 months. Any actual attempts at suicide or self-harm are rated according to method, physical condition after the attempt, and potential lethality of the attempt. Subjective reasons for the attempt are recorded as well as family response to the attempt. The subject is then asked what he or she feels are the chances that self-harm and/or a suicide attempt will occur within the next 6 months as well as at any time in the future. Lastly, the interviewer rates the subject on the suicidality scale, from 0 to 18,

ranging from "no suicidal ideation or self-destructive activity present or foreseeable" to "actively suicidal at present; would make life-endangering attempt given the opportunity."

Self-report measures included the following:

1. The Social Adjustment Scale—Self-Report (SAS-SR; Weissman and Bothwell 1976) covers a broad spectrum of social functioning, such as social and leisure activities, relationship with extended family, marital and parental roles, family unity, and economic independence. The SAS-SR has been shown to discriminate between psychiatric populations and healthy control subjects (Weissman et al. 1978).
2. Two self-report measures that have been discussed previously were used to measure impulsivity/aggression. The BDHI has a test–retest reliability ranging from .64 to .82 (Biaggio et al. 1981). We feel that the BDHI can be used to develop a global impression of angry and hostile feelings. In this study we report the BDHI subscale scores, the total BDHI score, and the BDHI emotion (attitudinal) factor and motor factors (Buss and Durkee 1957). The Barratt Impulsivity Scale—10th Revision (BIS-10; Barratt 1990) has three subscales with alpha coefficients ranging from .89 to .92; the three subscales have an average correlation of .34 with each other. Barratt states that in general the results show that the BIS-10 has clinical utility and trait specificity (Barratt 1985).

Results

One hundred percent of the required data were obtained in 96.3% of all subjects seen. Three subjects refused to complete the self-reports.

To appreciate which of several measures of impulsivity (BDHI, BIS) best correlates with DIB impulse action subscale scores, Pearson correlations were performed between current DIB and DIB-R total scores as well as impulse action subscale scores and 16 "predictive" impulsivity measures derived from the BDHI, BIS, and SBQ (Tables 1–1 and 1–2). Because of multiple comparisons, a Bonferroni correction was performed (.05/16) that led us to consider only those correlations achieving a significance level of less than or equal to .003 as statistically significant. Visual inspection of the data revealed few gross differences in the size of correlations with the DIB versus with the DIB-R total scores or with the DIB versus with the DIB-R impulse action subscale scores. There appeared to be a trend toward higher correlations with the DIB-R versus with the DIB total scores. We will henceforth refer primarily to the DIB and to DIB impulse action subscale scores.

DIB impulse action scores correlated with BDHI resentment, suspicion, and irritability scores. This DIB subscale correlated with the BDHI emotion factor but did not correlate with the motor factor. Correlation with the total BDHI score was also statistically significant (Table 1–1). Similar magnitudes of correlations were found between the DIB impulse action score and all the subscales of the BIS except the cognitive subscale. The correlation of the DIB impulse action subscale score with the SBQ was the highest achieved ($R = .54$, $P < .001$) (Table 1–2).

Correlations of the total DIB score with the BDHI subscale scores followed a pattern similar to the correlations with the

Table 1–1. Pearson correlations of DIB(R) and impulse action functioning with BDHI impulsivity

Outcome measures	BDHI										
	T	E	R	S	G	A	IN	IR	N	V	M
DIB impulse action subscale	.40*	.42*	.44*	.35*	.31	.26	.01	.49*	.32	.13	.33
DIB-R impulse action subscale	.41	.43*	.46*	.36	.33	.25	.03	.50*	.33	.13	.34
DIB score	.58*	.64*	.60*	.53*	.55*	.34	.16	.57*	.26	.27	.45*
DIB-R score	.63*	.72*	.65*	.59*	.65*	.31	.21	.62*	.24	.28	.48*

Note. A = assault. BDHI = Buss-Durkee Hostility Inventory (Buss and Durkee 1957). DIB = Diagnostic Interview for Borderlines (Gunderson et al. 1981). DIB-R = Diagnostic Interview for Borderlines—Revised (Zanarini et al. 1989). DIB(R) = DIB + DIB-R. E = emotion factor. G = guilt. IN = indirect hostility. IR = irritability. M = motor factor. N = negativism. R = resentment. S = suspicion. T = total. V = verbal hostility.
*Maintained significance after Bonferroni correction ($P < .003$).

Table 1–2. Pearson correlations of DIB(R) and impulse action functioning with BIS and SBQ impulsivity

Outcome measures	BIS				SBQ
	T	NP	M	C	
DIB impulse action subscale	.48*	.40*	.52*	.20	.54*
DIB-R impulse action subscale	.49*	.40	.51*	.24	.54*
DIB score	.35	.17	.46*	.19	.64*
DIB-R score	.41	.19	.52*	.26	.65*

Note. C = cognitive. BIS = Barratt Impulsivity Scale (Barratt 1965). DIB = Diagnostic Interview for Borderlines (Gunderson et al. 1981). DIB-R = Diagnostic Interview for Borderlines—Revised (Zanarini et al. 1989). DIB(R) = DIB + DIB-R. M = motor. NP = nonplanning. SBQ = Suicidal Behaviors Questionnaire (Linehan 1983). T = total.
*Maintained significance after Bonferroni correction ($P < .003$).

impulse action subscale score, with even more emotion factor subscale correlations significant here. Of interest is that there was a significant correlation with the motor factor of the BDHI as well. The correlation of the BDHI emotion factor with the total DIB-R score was the highest found ($R = .72$) (Table 1–1).

The pattern of correlations between DIB total and BIS scores changed from the pattern observed with DIB impulse action subscale scores. Only the motor subscale showed a significant correlation ($R = .46$, $P < .001$). The correlations with SBQ remained significant ($R = .64, P < .001$).

To better appreciate which measure of impulsivity best predicts current functioning, a series of stepwise multiple regression analyses was performed (Table 1–3). Each outcome (i.e., current functioning) measure was analyzed twice: 1) for analysis A, predictor variables included the BDHI total, its emotion and motor factors, and its subscale scores; the BIS total and its subscale scores; and the SBQ; 2) for analysis B, only the BDHI and BIS subscale scores and the SBQ were included as predictor variables. The outcome measures included the GAS, the SAS-SR, the DIB, and the DIB-R.

No item entered into the equations for the GAS. Results for the remaining three outcome measures were reasonably consistent

Table 1–3. Stepwise multiple regression of DIB-R and social functioning with impulsivity

Outcome measure	Predictor variable	Multiple R^2	Change in R^2	F ratio	P
DIB—Analysis A	1. SBQ	.42	.42	29.18	<.001
	2. BDHI	.61	.20	20.00	<.001
DIB—Analysis B	1. SBQ	.42	.42	29.18	<.001
	2. BDHI—guilt	.56	.15	13.17	.001
	3. BDHI—verbal hostility	.62	.06	6.50	<.05
DIB-R—Analysis A	1. BDHI—emotion factor	.48	.48	38.17	<.001
	2. SBQ	.62	.14	14.74	<.001
	3. BIS—motor	.67	.05	6.16	<.05
DIB-R—Analysis B	1. SBQ	.42	.42	29.11	<.001
	2. BDHI—guilt	.62	.20	21.21	<.05
	3. BIS—motor	.67	.05	6.17	<.05
SAS-SR—Analysis A	1. BDHI—emotion factor	.53	.53	46.52	<.001
	2. SBQ	.69	.16	20.65	<.001
	3. BDHI—irritability	.74	.05	7.05	<.05
SAS-SR—Analysis B	1. SBQ	.47	.47	35.88	<.001
	2. BDHI—guilt	.69	.22	28.06	<.001
	3. BDHI—irritability	.76	.07	12.00	.001

Note. The predictor variables for analysis A were BDHI total, BDHI subscales, BDHI emotion and motor factors, BIS total, BIS subscales, and SBQ; those for analysis B were BDHI subscales, BIS subscales, and SBQ. BDHI = Buss-Durkee Hostility Inventory (Buss and Durkee 1957). BIS = Barratt Impulsivity Scale (Barratt 1965). DIB = Diagnostic Interview for Borderlines (Gunderson et al. 1981). DIB-R = Diagnostic Interview for Borderlines—Revised (Zanarini et al. 1989). SAS-SR = Social Adjustment Scale—Self-Report (Weissman and Bothwell 1976). SBQ = Suicidal Behaviors Questionnaire (Linehan 1983).

across analyses. When the total BDHI and BIS scores (including the BDHI emotion and motor factors, i.e, analysis A) were included, the SBQ and the BDHI emotion factor tended to load most strongly into the equation. The exception was the DIB, in which the total BDHI score, rather than the emotion factor, entered in. Final additional items entering into these equations were the BIS motor score for the DIB-R and the BDHI irritability subscale score for the SAS-SR.

Results for analysis B (excluding the total and factor scores) were also remarkably consistent across analyses. The SBQ and the BDHI guilt subscale score entered into each analysis first and second, respectively. The final items entered included the BDHI verbal hostility subscale score for the DIB, the BIS motor score for the DIB-R, and the BDHI irritability score for the SAS-SR.

The results were strong, with multiple R^2 ranging from .62 to .76. Significance levels for the first two items entering into each equation were consistently less than .001.

DISCUSSION

As we discussed in the introduction to this chapter, impulsivity appears to be a core feature of BPD. Although the concept of impulsivity appears primarily in the impulse action subscale of the DIB and DIB-R, it is also found throughout other subscales of the DIB (e.g., affective lability and irritability). It is not surprising, then, that correlations with measures of impulsivity increased when moving from the impulse action subscale score to the total DIB(R) score (i.e., DIB + DIB-R). This finding was consistent for all the non-DIB measures of impulsivity.

However, the magnitude of the correlations with the BIS nonplanning score, and thus with the BIS total score as well, decreased when moving from the DIB impulse action subscale score to the total DIB score. BIS nonplanning, then, is closely associated with the behaviors found in the DIB impulse action subscale but not with the behaviors/affects found in the remainder of the DIB. Items in the nonplanning subscale relate to present versus future orientation—that is, to planning for social changes, financial matters, and so forth.

In general, our results are supportive of Gardner et al.'s (1991) earlier work, which showed that BPD subjects differ from healthy control subjects on the BDHI emotion factor and on the BDHI irritability subscale score. Although our study is uncontrolled, the results reveal strong correlations among both the DIB(R) impulse action and total DIB(R) scores and the BDHI emotion factor; the subscales that make up the emotion factor (resentment, suspicion, and guilt); and the irritability subscale score. Visual examination of the items comprised in these subscale scores shows excellent face validity. For example, the resentment subscale contains items such as "Other people always seem to get the breaks" and "At times I feel I get a raw deal out of life" (Buss and Durkee 1957). Gardner et al.'s use of the word "anger" in describing BPD patients is thus not inappropriate: BPD patients show considerable hostile affects and a "readiness to explode" (Buss and Durkee 1957, irritability subscale) but, significantly, do not, in fact, "explode"—at least not in terms of verbal and indirect hostility as measured by the BDHI. Indeed, the only DIB correlations that were found with "motoric" impulsivity on the BDHI were with the irritability subscale.

It appears that BPD patients may express their anger more frequently through self-mutilative and suicidal thoughts and actions (as measured by the SBQ). Although motor impulsiveness, as measured by the BIS, did correlate with the DIB and its impulse action subscale, visual inspection of the items comprised in the BIS motor subscale reveals, in contrast to the BDHI motor subscale, a tendency to be restless, inattentive, and to act without anticipation of the consequences.

The BPD concept of impulse action, therefore (and, indeed, the global DIB concept of BPD), seems to correlate best with items related to irritable and angry affects, and (perhaps secondarily) to suicidality. The correlations with BIS motor impulsiveness are of interest; it is possible that the dispositions measured here—inattentiveness, restlessness, entering into actions without anticipation of consequences—point us toward a biological basis for anger, irritability, suicidality, and ultimately the BPD diagnosis. The items in the BIS motor subscale bear a striking resemblance to symptoms/behaviors shown in ADHD and in "frontal lobe syndromes," especially where there has been damage to the orbital frontal cortex (Cummings 1985). Andrulonis and Vogel (1984) found a strong association between BPD and ADHD, traumatic brain injury, and various other CNS lesions, a finding we have been able to replicate (van Reekum et al. 1993). Perhaps some subtle or not-so-subtle brain dysfunction leads to inattention/restlessness and to action without anticipation. If the future borderline adult struggles during childhood with these predispositions, we can appreciate how repeated academic/vocational and interpersonal failures could lead secondarily to angry/irritable affects and a tendency to self-harm.

Despite the evidence presented by deVegvar et al. in Chapter 2, our results do not strongly support an etiological relationship between impulsivity and low CNS serotonergic activity. Whereas irritability is strongly associated with both impulse action (and total DIB) scores and measures of low CNS serotonergic activity (Coccaro et al. 1989), the most strongly associated element of impulsivity in our BPD sample—the BDHI emotion factor—has not been found to be associated with low CNS serotonergic activity (Coccaro et al. 1989). Low CNS serotonergic activity appears to be related to the "readiness to explode" (i.e., irritability on the BDHI, which was found to be associated with BPD in this study), as well as to the tendency to actually explode (i.e., assaultiveness on the BDHI, which was not associated with BPD in this study).

Results from the stepwise multiple regression analyses reveal that certain measures of impulsivity, collected cross-sectionally, could explain much (up to 76%) of the variance in current BPD diagnosis (DIB and DIB-R scores) and current social functioning (SAS-SR). The corollary here is that many measures of impulsivity consistently did not enter into the equations. The BDHI emotion factor was the strongest predictor of current functioning as defined by the DIB-R and the SAS-SR when it was included in the analysis. The SBQ entered into these equations very strongly, and indeed was the strongest predictor of the current DIB score. The BDHI emotion factor was replaced by the total BDHI score in the equation predicting the DIB. In summary, the BDHI emotion factor and the SBQ appear to strongly "predict" current BPD diagnosis and social functioning.

SUMMARY AND CONCLUSIONS

The studies reviewed and data presented here strongly suggest that impulsivity is a central feature of BPD. However, it is also clear that the term *impulsivity*, although used widely, lacks precision. In BPD at least, this term may be replaced by the terms *anger* (which can be used to summarize the BDHI emotion factor), *suicidality*, and *irritability*. These three terms correlated highly with DIB and DIB-R total scores and with impulse action subscale scores in our sample of BPD patients.

Whereas other impulsivity measures also correlated highly with the DIB measures, the strongest predictors of current BPD diagnosis, as well as of current social functioning, were consistently the SBQ (suicidality) and the BDHI emotion factor. Targeting treatment interventions toward these elements of impulsivity would seem appropriate.

Results from this study also suggest the hypothesis that inattentiveness and a tendency toward action without anticipation of the consequences (BIS motor) may underlie a substantial portion of the "impulsivity" seen in BPD. These behaviors may be linked to brain disorders such as ADHD and traumatic brain injury.

A few notes of caution should be mentioned. The original research presented here suffers from a lack of *a priori* hypotheses; future replication studies are required. Further, "outcome" here is defined cross-sectionally, and we have studied the ability of impulsivity measures to "predict" current functioning. We hope to assess the ability of impulsivity to predict long-term (as opposed to current) outcome in future follow-up studies with this cohort.

REFERENCES

American Psychiatric Association: Diagnostic and Statistical Manual of Mental Disorders, 3rd Edition. Washington, DC, American Psychiatric Association, 1980

American Psychiatric Association: Diagnostic and Statistical Manual of Mental Disorders, 3rd Edition, Revised. Washington, DC, American Psychiatric Association, 1987

Andrulonis PA, Vogel NG: Comparison of borderline personality subcategories to schizophrenic and affective disorders. Br J Psychiatry 144:358–363, 1984

Barratt ES: Factor analysis of some psychometric measures of impulsiveness and anxiety. Psychol Rep 16:547–554, 1965

Barratt ES: Impulsiveness subtraits: arousal and information processing, in Motivation, Emotion and Personality: Proceedings of the 23rd International Congress of Psychology, Vol 5. Amsterdam, Elsevier, 1985, pp 137–146

Barratt ES: Impulsiveness and aggression. Paper presented at the Risk Special Studies Meeting, McArthur Foundation Program of Research on Mental Health and Behavior, Pittsburgh, PA, September 1990

Biaggio M, Supplee K, Curtis N: Reliability and validity of four anger scales. J Pers Assess 45:639–648, 1981

Brown GL, Goodwin FK, Ballenger JC, et al: Aggression in humans: correlates with cerebrospinal fluid amine metabolites. Psychiatry Res 1:131–139, 1979

Burgess JW: Relationship of depression and cognitive impairment to self-injury in borderline personality disorder, major depression, and schizophrenia. Psychiatry Res 38:77–87, 1991

Buss AH, Durkee A: An inventory for assessing different kinds of hostility. Journal of Consulting Psychology 21:343–349, 1957

Coccaro EF, Siever LJ, Klar HM, et al: Serotonergic studies in patients with affective and personality disorders: correlates with suicidal and impulsive aggressive behavior. Arch Gen Psychiatry 46:587–599, 1989

Coccaro EF, Harvey PD, Kupsaw-Lawrence E, et al: Development of neuropharmacologically based behavioral assessments of impulsive aggressive behavior. J Neuropsychiatry Clin Neurosci 3:S44–S50, 1991

Cornelius JR, Soloff PH, Perel JM, et al: Fluoxetine trial in borderline personality disorder. Psychopharmacol Bull 26:151–154, 1990

Cowdry RW, Gardner DL: Pharmacotherapy of borderline personality disorder: alprazolam, carbamazepine, trifluoperazine and tranylcypromine. Arch Gen Psychiatry 45:111–119, 1988

Cummings JL: Clinical Neuropsychiatry. Orlando, FL, Grune & Stratton, 1985

Derogatis LR, Lipman RS, Covi L: SCL-90: an outpatient psychiatric rating scale—preliminary report. Psychopharmacol Bull 9:13–28, 1973

Endicott J, Spitzer R, Fleiss J, et al: The global assessment scale: a procedure for measuring overall severity of psychiatric disturbance. Arch Gen Psychiatry 33:766–771, 1976

Gardner DL, Lucas PB, Cowdry CW: CSF metabolites in borderline personality disorder compared with normal controls. Biol Psychiatry 28:247–254, 1990

Gardner DL, Leibenluft E, O'Leary K, et al: Self-ratings of anger and hostility in borderline personality disorder. J Nerv Ment Dis 179:157–161, 1991

Gunderson JG, Phillips KA: A current view of the interface between borderline personality disorder and depression. Am J Psychiatry 148:967–975, 1991

Gunderson JG, Zanarini MC: Pathogenesis of borderline personality, in American Psychiatric Press Review of Psychiatry, Vol 8. Edited by Tasman A, Hales RE, Frances AJ. Washington, DC, American Psychiatric Press, 1989, pp 25–49

Gunderson JG, Carpenter WT, Strauss JS: Borderline and schizophrenic patients: a comparative study. Am J Psychiatry 132:1257–1264, 1975

Gunderson JG, Kolb JE, Austin V: The Diagnostic Interview for Borderline Patients. Am J Psychiatry 138:896–903, 1981

Kernberg O: Borderline Conditions and Pathological Narcissism. New York, Jason Aronson, 1975

Kernberg O: Object Relations Theory and Clinical Psychoanalysis. New York, Jason Aronson, 1976

Kotila L, Lonnquist J: Adolescents who make suicide attempts repeatedly. Acta Psychiatr Scand 76:386–393, 1987

Linehan MM: Suicidal Behaviors Questionnaire. Seattle, WA, University of Washington, 1983

Linehan MM, Armstrong HE, Suarez A, et al: Cognitive-behavioral treatment of chronically parasuicidal borderline patients. Arch Gen Psychiatry 48:1060–1064, 1991

Links PS, Boiago I: Borderline as impulse disorder: family evidence. Paper presented at the 143rd annual meeting of the American Psychiatric Association, New York, May 1990

Links PS, Steiner M, Boiago I, et al: Lithium therapy for borderline patients: preliminary findings. Journal of Personality Disorders 4:173–181, 1990a

Links PS, Mitton JE, Steiner M: Predicting outcome for borderline personality disorder. Compr Psychiatry 31:490–498, 1990b

Markovitz PJ, Calabrese JR, Schulz CR, et al: Fluoxetine in the treatment of borderline and schizotypal personality disorders. Am J Psychiatry 148:1064–1067, 1991

McGlashan TH: The Chestnut Lodge follow-up study, I: follow-up methodology and study sample. Arch Gen Psychiatry 41:573–585, 1984

McGlashan TH: The prediction of outcome in borderline personality disorder: part V of the Chestnut Lodge follow-up study, in The Borderline: Current Empirical Research. Edited by McGlashan TH. Washington, DC, American Psychiatric Press, 1985, pp 61–98

Norden MJ: Fluoxetine in borderline personality disorder. Prog Neuropsychopharmacol Biol Psychiatry 13:885–893, 1989

Paris J, Brown R, Nowliss D: Long-term follow-up of borderline patients in a general hospital. Compr Psychiatry 28:530–535, 1987

Perry JC, Klerman GL: Clinical features of the borderline personality disorder. Am J Psychiatry 137:165–173, 1980

Pfohl B, Blum N, Zimmerman M, et al: Structured Interview for DSM-III-R Personality Disorders (SIDP-R). Iowa City, IA, University of Iowa College of Medicine, Department of Psychiatry, 1989

Soloff PH: Affect, impulse and psychosis in borderline disorders: a validation study. Compr Psychiatry 22:337–350, 1981a

Soloff PH: Concurrent validation of a diagnostic interview for borderline patients. Am J Psychiatry 138:691–693, 1981b

Soloff PH, George A, Nathan RS, et al: Progress in the pharmacotherapy of borderline disorders. Arch Gen Psychiatry 43:691–697, 1986

Soloff PH, George A, Nathan RS, et al: Amitriptyline vs. haloperidol in borderlines. Paper presented at the 140th annual meeting of the American Psychiatric Association, Chicago, IL, May 1987

Stone MH, Hurt SW, Stone DK: The P.I.-500: long-term follow-up of borderline patients meeting DSM-III criteria, I: global outcome. Journal of Personality Disorders 1:291–298, 1988

Stone MH: The course of borderline personality disorder, in American Psychiatric Press Review of Psychiatry, Vol 8. Edited by Tasman A, Hales RE, Frances AJ. Washington, DC, American Psychiatric Press, 1989, pp 103–122

van Reekum R, Conway C, Gansler D, et al: Neurobehavioral study of borderline personality disorder. J Psychiatry Neurosci 18:121–129, 1993

Weissman MM, Bothwell S: Assessment of social adjustment by patient self-report. Arch Gen Psychiatry 33:1111–1115, 1976

Weissman MM, Prusoff B, Thompson M, et al: Social adjustment by self-report in a community sample and in psychiatric outpatients. J Nerv Ment Dis 166:317–326, 1978

Zanarini MC, Gunderson JG, Frankenburg FR, et al: The revised diagnostic interview for borderlines: discriminating BPD from other Axis II disorders. Journal of Personality Disorders 3:10–18, 1989

Chapter 2

Impulsivity and Serotonin in Borderline Personality Disorder

Marie-Louise deVegvar, M.D.
Larry J. Siever, M.D.
Robert L. Trestman, M.D., Ph.D.

The DSM-III-R (American Psychiatric Association 1987) diagnosis of borderline personality disorder (BPD) is defined as "a pervasive pattern of instability of mood, interpersonal relationships, and self-image" and is characterized by criteria that include potentially self-damaging impulsivity, inappropriate or uncontrolled anger, recurrent suicidal threats or gestures, and physically self-damaging acts (p. 347). Impulsivity/aggression is also characteristic of other personality disorders in what has become known as Cluster B (the dramatic cluster), which consists of the histrionic, narcissistic, antisocial, and borderline personality disorders. However, impulsivity/aggression may be expressed somewhat differently in each disorder (American Psychiatric Association 1987). For example, in antisocial personality disorder, coupled with impulsivity/aggression is a disregard for social norms that leads to behaviors such as lying, stealing, and destroying property. In the histrionic patient, impulsivity/aggression may play a part in low frustration tolerance, and in the narcissistic patient it may be involved in the patient's rage in response to criticism. This suggests, then, that impulsivity/aggression can be considered a dimension of behavior that is not restricted to a single psychiatric diagnosis and that may occur in Axis I (i.e., intermittent explosive disorder; bipolar disorder, manic type; and conduct disorder) as well as Axis II disorders (Siever and Davis 1991). (Impulsivity/aggression is combined here into one symptom, criterion, or dimension because it appears that aggression—whether against self, others, or property—is one of the most troubling behavioral manifestations of impulsive behavior.)

A vulnerability to impulsivity/aggression suggests a dysregulation of systems responsible for modulating and inhibiting aggressive behaviors in response to environmental cues. Serotonin (5-hydroxytryptamine [5-HT]) is generally thought to be a modulatory neurotransmitter with inhibitory effects. Serotonin plays a role in a number of central nervous system (CNS)–mediated functions, including mood, sleep, arousal, sexual activity, feeding behavior, cognition, and neuroendocrine function (Siever et al. 1991).

Animal studies demonstrate that lesions of the serotonergic system may produce a lack of extinction of punished behaviors and may also disinhibit aggression. The association between diminished serotonergic function and unrestrained aggression is also seen in a number of other studies that use a variety of indices to assess serotonergic function. These studies, which include human autopsy studies of receptors and metabolites, studies of 5-hydroxyindoleacetic acid (5-HIAA) in cerebrospinal fluid (CSF), examinations of platelet imipramine binding and receptor sites, and neuroendocrine challenge studies, are outlined in Table 2–1. In this chapter we explore in more detail the basic, preclinical, and clinical evidence that suggests that disturbances in the serotonergic system play a role in impulsivity/aggression in BPD and perhaps in other personality disorders as well.

ANIMAL STUDIES AND AGGRESSION

Many studies have shown that aggressive behavior in animals is decreased by drugs that increase serotonergic function. Kostowski and colleagues (1984) found that fluoxetine suppressed muricidal (killing of mice by rats or cats) behavior in rats at doses that produced no sedation or other obvious behavioral effects. Not only has fluoxetine been shown to decrease sponta-

Table 2–1. Indices of serotonin (5-HT)

Index	Information
Metabolites	
Cerebrospinal fluid 5-hydroxyindoleacetic acid (5-HIAA)	The main metabolite of 5-HT; putatively, a measure of central, presynaptic 5-HT turnover
Binding studies	
Platelet 5-HT uptake	A measure of peripheral uptake sites that might parallel central presynaptic function
Platelet imipramine binding	Related to the peripheral 5-HT uptake site; a measure that may parallel central 5-HT presynaptic function
Platelet 5-HT$_2$ binding	A putative postsynaptic measure of a specific 5-HT receptor subtype (5-HT$_2$); measures are activity (K_d) and number (B_{max})
Brain imipramine binding	Related to 5-HT uptake site; a putative measure of 5-HT presynaptic function
Brain 5-HT$_2$ receptor binding	A postsynaptic measure of a specific 5-HT receptor subtype (5-HT$_2$); measures are activity (K_d), number (B_{max}), and distribution
Challenge studies	
Fenfluramine	A 5-HT–releasing, uptake-inhibiting, and postsynaptic stimulating agent; the plasma prolactin response provides a "net" measure of overall pre- and postsynaptic 5-HT function
m-Chlorophenylpiperazine (m-CPP)	A 5-HT postsynaptic receptor agonist that works primarily at 5-HT$_{1C}$, 5-HT$_2$, and 5-HT$_3$ receptor sites; the plasma prolactin response provides a partially selective measure of postsynaptic 5-HT function
Buspirone	A selective 5-HT$_{1A}$ agonist; the plasma prolactin response provides a selective measure of postsynaptic 5-HT$_{1A}$ function

neous muricidal behavior in rats, it also reversed rats' muricidal behavior that had been induced by olfactory bulb ablation, social isolation, and electrolytic lesions of raphe nuclei, all of which can inhibit synthesis of serotonin (Kostowski et al. 1984; Molina et al. 1987; Stark et al. 1985). These results suggest that deficits in serotonin may lead to increased aggression.

AUTOPSY STUDIES

Postmortem studies have been undertaken to measure serotonin receptors and to assess the brain serotonergic system. Arango and colleagues (1990), in a study of 11 suicide victims and 11 matched control subjects, examined membrane binding and quantitative receptor autoradiography of $5\text{-}HT_2$ receptor binding sites. They found a significant increase in the $5\text{-}HT_2$ receptor binding sites in suicide victims across all cortical layers in the prefrontal cortex. The cause of this increase in $5\text{-}HT_2$ receptors is not known, although one could speculate that it is associated with reduced serotonin release. However, animal studies have looked at the effect of decreased serotonin release secondary to lesions of the brain stem raphe nuclei; results of these studies are inconsistent with regard to demonstrating upregulation, or an increase in the number, of postsynaptic $5\text{-}HT_2$ receptors (Mann and Arango 1992). Although these results are not conclusive, they do suggest a role for serotonin in the regulation of self-directed aggression (i.e., suicide), and support for this role for serotonin, as will be discussed later, has been found in clinical studies of patients with personality disorders who have impulsive aggressive behavior.

CSF 5-HIAA

Measurement of CSF concentrations of 5-HT and 5-HIAA is another approach that has been applied to the study of the relationship of serotonergic function to aggressive impulsive behavior and suicide. Over the past decade, many research reports have described decreased CSF 5-HIAA in different clinical and nonclinical populations, all with the common characteristic of having violent and/or impulsive behaviors. Reduced concentrations of CSF 5-HIAA have been correlated with a lifetime history of physical aggression toward others and high scores of psychopathic deviance as assessed by the Minnesota Multiphasic Personality Inventory (MMPI; G. L. Brown et al. 1982). Within some of these groups, the degree and nature of the violent behavior was related to CSF 5-HIAA. For example, Linnoila et al. (1983), in a study of violent offenders with DSM-III (American Psychiatric Association 1980) personality disorders and alcoholism, found that CSF 5-HIAA levels were significantly lower in 27 violent offenders whose crimes were assessed as "impulsive" than in 9 nonviolent offenders whose crimes were assessed to have been premeditated. Further, offenders who had committed more than one violent crime had lower CSF 5-HIAA levels than offenders with a record of only one violent crime. A decrease in CSF 5-HIAA was also noted among people who had murdered their own children (Lidberg et al. 1984) as well as among murderers with depression, anxiety, and personality disorders (Lidberg et al. 1985) and among arsonists (Virkkunen et al. 1987). Recently, Kruesi and colleagues (1990) observed lower CSF 5-HIAA levels in children and adolescents with disruptive behavior disorders when compared with age-, sex-, and race-matched children with obsessive-compulsive disorder.

In addition to violence against others, decreased concentrations of CSF 5-HIAA have been reported in suicidal patients, regardless of their psychiatric diagnosis. Åsberg et al. (1976) studied CSF 5-HIAA concentrations in hospitalized, medication-free, depressed patients; those patients with histories of violent suicidal behavior had significantly lower CSF 5-HIAA concentrations than patients with more benign, non-self-destructive histories. Åsberg et al. (1976) also found lower concentrations of CSF 5-HIAA in a diagnostically mixed group of hospitalized patients with histories of suicidal behavior when compared with patients without histories of suicidality. G. L. Brown and colleagues (1982) found that 12 BPD patients without major depression had histories of aggressive behavior and suicide attempts that were significantly associated with each other; further, each of these behaviors (aggression and suicidality) was also independently associated with lower CSF 5-HIAA levels.

In patients with a primary diagnosis of major depression, low CSF 5-HIAA concentrations are associated with suicidality but not with depression per se (see review by Siever et al. 1991). A similar finding has been reported among elderly, depressed, suicidal patients, who were found to have lower concentrations of CSF 5-HIAA than either elderly, depressed patients who were not suicidal or age-matched nonpsychiatrically ill control subjects (Jones et al. 1990). A separate 5-year follow-up study reported that depressed patients who reattempted suicide had significantly lower CSF 5-HIAA concentrations than depressed patients who either had never attempted or had not reattempted suicide (Roy et al. 1989).

Studies of CSF 5-HIAA have an inherent limitation: they are a static measure of presynaptic CNS serotonergic activity only and do not reflect "net" serotonergic activity. However, these studies do lend support to the hypothesis that there is a correlation between decreased serotonergic activity and increased impulsive aggression toward self and/or others. This relationship can be particularly applicable to patients with personality disorders, especially those personality disorders in which impulsiveness and aggression are important components of the clinical picture and of the interpersonal dysfunction (e.g., BPD).

PLATELET MEASURES OF SEROTONIN

Platelets may also be studied as possible models for CNS serotonergic function. In an examination of serotonin uptake in platelets, 15 male patients with "episodic aggression" were compared with age- and sex-matched control subjects (C. S. Brown et al. 1989). Lower mean 5-HT uptake was found in the platelets of the aggressive patients, a finding consistent with the hypothesis that reduced platelet 5-HT uptake reflects reduced CNS 5-HT function. In the same study, there was a significant negative correlation between 5-HT uptake and impulsivity (C. S. Brown et al. 1989). Correlations between low platelet 5-HT uptake and aggressive behavior have been found among schizophrenic adolescents as well (Modai et al. 1989).

Marazziti et al. (1989) compared the tritiated imipramine-binding parameters of platelets in a group of female suicide attempters and a group of control subjects. The receptor number, or B_{max}, was found to be significantly lower in suicide attempters when compared with nonpsychiatrically ill control subjects; this "lowering" of the number of receptors appeared to occur without modification of the function of the receptor, since the dissociation constant, K_d, remained unchanged. Meltzer and Arora (1986) reported that platelet monoamine oxidase (MAO) activity and the K_d of platelet imipramine binding were significant predictors of ratings of suicide on the Hamilton Rating Scale for Depression (Hamilton 1960). Other researchers have found platelet 5-HT$_2$ receptors to be increased in suicidal patients when compared with nonsuicidal patients and control subjects (Pandey et al. 1990). It should be noted that in these studies, as in the studies of CSF 5-HIAA, platelet measures of serotonin reflect only presynaptic serotonergic function and therefore provide us with an incomplete picture of "net" serotonergic activity. However, the findings in these platelet studies are consistent with the findings in autopsy and CSF studies in supporting the correlation between increased impulsive aggression toward self and/or others and decreased serotonergic function.

CHALLENGE STUDIES AS A MEASURE OF SEROTONERGIC DISTURBANCE

Neuroendocrine challenge studies offer a means of assessing the functional responsivity of CNS serotonergic systems. Challenge studies can be accomplished by administering serotonergic agents to research subjects. After the administration of serotonergic agents, the changes found in plasma concentration of specific hormones whose release is regulated, at least in part, by serotonin, are then measured. Secretion of these specific hormones is thought to be linked to stimulation of 5-HT receptors on hypothalamic cells by the serotonergic agents. Hypothalamic-releasing factors then act on targeted anterior pituitary cells, which in turn secrete the hormone—in this case, prolactin (PRL) and/or adrenocorticotropic hormone (ACTH) (Coccaro et al. 1990b). For example, the release of PRL in response to the administration of fenfluramine, a 5-HT releasing/uptake inhibiting agent, is blocked by lesions of the raphe nuclei and by pretreatment with 5-HT antagonists, and the PRL response to fenfluramine is dose related (Coccaro et al. 1989). Although fenfluramine's inhibiting actions are presynaptic, they may also reflect postsynaptic responsivity through the effects of fenfluramine's active metabolite norfenfluramine, which has direct postsynaptic stimulatory effects (Coccaro et al. 1989). We may therefore be able to assess the overall effect of pre- and postsynaptic actions of CNS 5-HT function by employing a challenge with fenfluramine.

Coccaro and associates (1989) examined the PRL response to fenfluramine in 45 male patients with affective disorder and/or personality disorder and in 18 male control subjects. PRL responses to fenfluramine among all the patients were reduced compared with those of the controls. Reduced PRL responses were correlated with impulsive aggression only in the personality disorder patients; there was no correlation of the PRL response with depression. Significant negative correlations were found in the patients for whom personality disorder was the primary diagnosis. These correlations were found between the reduced PRL response to fenfluramine and the "assault" and "irritability" subscales of the Buss-Durkee Hostility Inventory (BDHI; Buss and Durkee 1957) and the "motor behavior" subscale of the Barratt Impulsivity Scale (BIS; Barratt and Patton 1983). (These scales are discussed in more detail in Chapter 1.) Further, the patients who met DSM-III criteria for borderline personality disorder ($n = 8$) had significantly reduced change in peak PRL response (delta PRL response) to fenfluramine compared with both the patients without BPD ($n = 12$) and the control subjects of a similar age range ($n = 14$). Coccaro et al. (1989) also found that whereas a reduced PRL response to fenfluramine correlated with a history of suicide attempts in all of the depressed patients as well as the personality disorder patients, the reduced PRL response correlated (inversely) with clinician and self-reported ratings of impulsive aggression only in the personality disorder patients.

The above study was extended to include a larger sample ($n = 33$) and a second hospital. Results of the extended study were consistent with the original study (Trestman et al. 1992b). In the extended study, the results demonstrated a negative correlation in male subjects between the PRL response to fenfluramine and measures of impulsivity and aggression ($n = 32$; BIS–motor impulsivity: $r = -.34$, $P < .03$; BDHI–assault: $r = -.56$, $P < .001$). This larger sample of BPD patients also showed a blunted delta PRL response to fenfluramine when compared with non-BPD patients. The delta PRL of the personality disorder subjects who met the individual impulsive/aggressive criteria of BPD continued to be significantly lower than that of the patients who did not meet these criteria.

Preliminary studies from our laboratory have extended these original studies to include an examination of other neurotransmitters that also have the potential of contributing to aggression, impulsivity, and suicidality in patients. The noradrenergic system is involved in the engagement of the person with his or her environment, and it would, therefore, be a system that could be fruitful to examine. (The noradrenergic system is discussed in more detail in Chapter 3.) The noradrenergic system involves norepinephrine and has two classes of receptors: alpha and beta. These receptors are further subdivided into $alpha_1$, $alpha_2$, $beta_1$, and $beta_2$. $Alpha_1$ receptors are postsynaptic, $alpha_2$ receptors are presynaptic and postsynaptic, and both beta receptors are postsynaptic. There is evidence that presynaptic receptors play a role in the modulation of norepinephrine release in norepinephrine neurons. Several of the presynaptic receptors (i.e., $alpha_2$-adrenergic receptors) are involved in the inhibition of norepinephrine release from adrenergic neurons. Clonidine is an $alpha_2$-adrenergic agonist and stimulates presynaptic $alpha_2$ receptors to inhibit norepinephrine release (Cooper et al. 1991). In animals, the growth hormone response to clonidine is blocked by yohimbine, an $alpha_2$-adrenergic antagonist, and clonidine may therefore be used as a neuroendocrine challenge within the noradrenergic system (Siever et al. 1992).

Serotonergic function was assessed in 39 personality disorder patients by measuring CSF 5-HIAA as well as the PRL response to fenfluramine (Trestman et al. 1992a). CNS noradrenergic function was assessed by measuring basal plasma norepinephrine and the 60-minute growth hormone response to clonidine. Impulsive aggressive behavior was measured with the BDHI and the BIS. The results demonstrated a correlation between growth hormone response to clonidine and self-rated measures of irritability ($n = 39$; BDHI–irritability: $r = .28$, $P < .07$; BDHI–verbal hostility: $r = .37$, $P < .03$), but there was no correlation between the growth hormone response and violence or a history of suicidal behavior. In addition, increased basal plasma norepinephrine correlated with measures of impulsive risk taking. No correlation was found between CSF 5-HIAA and measures of impulsive aggressive behavior, in contrast with the findings of other studies of CSF 5-HIAA discussed previously. There was, however, a significant negative correlation between the PRL response to fenfluramine and CSF 5-HIAA ($n = 18$, $r = -.47$, $P < .05$). This latter result suggests that an abnormality of a serotonergic receptor subtype might cause an increase in presynaptic 5-HT activity, as reflected by CSF 5-HIAA concentrations, but more studies will be needed to further clarify the relationship between pre- and postsynaptic indices. These findings also suggest a role for the noradrenergic system in the modulation of impulsive and aggressive behaviors. Specifically, increased noradrenergic activity may indicate an abnormally heightened reactivity to the environment, since increased noradrenergic activity is correlated with increased irritability but not with physical acts of aggression (this idea is elaborated further in Chapter 3).

Further evidence of a relationship between impulsive aggressive behavior and serotonergic function has been found in a preliminary family study (Coccaro et al. 1994). This family study examined the risk of impulsive aggression, affective instability, and cognitive/perceptual distortions in 76 first-degree relatives of 18 male patients who had a primary diagnosis of personality disorder and who had undergone the fenfluramine challenge test. Family history diagnoses were assessed using the Family History Research Diagnostic Criteria (Andreasen et al. 1977) and additional family history criteria for affective, impulsive, and schizophrenia-related personality disorder traits (criteria are available from the authors upon request). The results reveal that the risk of impulsive personality disorder traits are significantly increased in the relatives of those probands with reduced PRL responses to fenfluramine. However, high scores on indices of impulsive aggression in the probands do not correlate with an increased risk for impulsive personality disorder traits in the relatives. This suggests that the first-degree relatives of probands with a CNS 5-HT abnormality are at increased risk for impulsive aggression, and measures of serotonergic function in patients may be a more sensitive indicator of this familial trait than the behaviors themselves.

Buspirone is another agent that can be employed in neuroendocrine challenges. Buspirone is a nonbenzodiazepine anxiolytic and a 5-HT_{1A} agonist that stimulates the release of both cortisol and PRL. Pretreatment with metergoline, a nonselective 5-HT receptor antagonist, blocks the response of PRL to buspirone (Coccaro et al. 1990a). Pindolol is a nonselective beta-adrenergic antagonist and a 5-HT_{1A} mixed agonist-antagonist that at a dose of 20 mg suppresses the PRL but not the cortisol response to buspirone (Coccaro et al. 1990a). However, at a dose of 30 mg, pindolol has no effect on the PRL response to buspirone. This suggests that doses of pindolol greater than 20 mg block the 5-HT_{1A} receptors mediating PRL release much less effectively than lower doses.

A preliminary study examined the PRL response to buspirone in 5 male volunteers and 10 male and female patients with personality disorders (Coccaro et al. 1990a). In the patients, there was a negative correlation between the PRL response to buspirone and self-assessed "irritability" as measured on the BDHI. This further supports the inverse relationship between impulsive aggression and serotonergic function and suggests that it may be partially modulated by postsynaptic 5-HT_{1A} receptors.

A limitation of the majority of these studies done by our group is their predominant focus on men, particularly since it is thought that two-thirds of patients with BPD are women (Vaillant and Perry 1985). Possible gender differences in serotonergic function need to be examined.

GENDER DIFFERENCES IN SEROTONERGIC MECHANISMS

Observable gender differences have been found in several serotonin-modulated behaviors, such as aggression and impulsivity

(Buss and Durkee 1957; Dietz 1987; Kellermann and Mercy 1992). Men demonstrate four times the lethal violence of women (Kellermann and Mercy 1992), whereas women are more prone to verbal and indirect forms of aggression than are men (Buss and Durkee 1957). These findings raise the possibility of gender-related differences in serotonergic mechanisms in the brain (Lepage and Steiner 1991).

Animal studies have demonstrated higher brain levels of serotonin in female mammals compared with male mammals (Carlsson and Carlsson 1988) and increased imipramine binding in the whole brains of female rats compared with male rats (Ieni et al. 1985). Compared with male rats, female rats evidenced a greater increase in brain serotonin and 5-HIAA following administration of inescapable shock in two different paradigms (Heinsbroek et al. 1990). Further, female mammals demonstrate greater responsiveness to pharmacological intervention with serotonergic agents (O'Connor and Feder 1985) and show less serotonin depletion–induced aggression (Valzelli et al. 1981) than do male mammals. Arato and associates (1991) used tritiated imipramine-binding sites to study the orbital frontal cortex in six men and women; these researchers reported significant interhemispheric asymmetry in both sexes, with a higher B_{max} on the right side than on the left. Also, the women had higher B_{max} values in imipramine binding in the right orbital frontal cortex than did the men.

Charney et al. (1988) used m-chlorophenylpiperazine, a serotonin receptor agonist, to compare male and female patients with obsessive-compulsive disorder with control subjects. A significant reduction in PRL response and lower baseline PRL levels were observed in the female obsessive-compulsive disorder patients compared with the female control subjects; there were no differences in the PRL responses and baseline PRL levels of the male obsessive-compulsive disorder patients and those of the male volunteer subjects. Overall, these data suggest that there are specific gender differences in the CNS serotonergic system.

In summary, then, these studies are consistent with a hypothesis of gender-differentiated serotonergic involvement in the control of impulsivity and aggression.

IMPLICATIONS FOR PHARMACOLOGICAL TREATMENT

As we have shown in this chapter, there is growing evidence of a biological contribution to impulsive aggressive behaviors, and this biological underpinning to impulsive aggression raises the possibility that pharmacological agents may have a role in the treatment of these disorders. Pharmacological implications of the studies in this volume are discussed in Chapter 11. Briefly, lithium has been shown to reduce physically aggressive behavior in a group of prison inmates (Sheard et al. 1976), although the mechanism of action is not clear. Lithium enhances postsynaptic serotonergic receptor function and may also decrease catecholaminergic function (Linnoila et al. 1983). Therefore, the antiaggressive property of lithium may be due to its serotonergic activity, its effect on catecholaminergic activity, or some dynamic interaction between these two systems (Coccaro et al. 1990a).

A preliminary pharmacological study demonstrated the ability of the serotonin reuptake blocker fluoxetine to diminish impulsive behaviors in patients with BPD (Norden 1989). Another preliminary pharmacological study revealed that buspirone may be effective in reducing aggression in a group of patients with mental retardation (Ratey et al. 1991). Nonselective beta-blockers such as propranolol have also been reported to decrease aggressive behavior in patients with organic brain damage (Yudofsky et al. 1981). This suggests that multiple mechanisms may be involved in the modulation of impulsive aggression, although there may well be significant differences between patients who exhibit impulsive aggressive behavior secondary to a personality disorder such as BPD and those who exhibit aggression and impulsivity as the result of an organic brain syndrome.

CONCLUSIONS

Impulsive aggressive behavior is a dimensional characteristic that may occur in individuals across a number of psychiatric diagnoses, although it is particularly common in patients with borderline and/or antisocial personality disorders. A series of studies supports the hypothesis that dysregulation of the CNS serotonergic system is related to impulsive aggression toward self or others. These studies have methodological limitations because there currently is no ideal method for assessing CNS serotonergic function. Animal models are simplistic and have restricted applicability to human behavior; results of postmortem studies are inconsistent, in part due to methodology; and clinical studies also have limitations, because they make assumptions and inferences about the actual workings of CNS mechanisms. For example, CSF 5-HIAA concentrations reflect only presynaptic serotonergic function, whereas neuroendocrine challenge paradigms may reflect "net" CNS serotonergic function but have limited specificity. In the future, neuroimaging studies of the functioning human brain using 5-HT–specific ligands might address some of these limitations and provide an opportunity to study the dynamic activity of the CNS serotonergic system (see Chapter 6 for a more detailed discussion of the uses of neuroimaging in the personality disorders). Understanding the differential neurophysiological contributions to any specific behavior of the serotonergic and noradrenergic systems (among others) may provide additional insights to help guide the development of psychopharmacological agents that may eventually provide better management of problematic and potentially lethal behaviors.

REFERENCES

American Psychiatric Association: Diagnostic and Statistical Manual of Mental Disorders, 3rd Edition. Washington DC, American Psychiatric Association, 1980

American Psychiatric Association: Diagnostic and Statistical Manual of Mental Disorders, 3rd Edition, Revised. Washington DC, American Psychiatric Association, 1987

Andreasen NC, Endicott J, Spitzer RL, et al: The family history method using diagnostic criteria: reliability and validity. Arch Gen Psychiatry 34:1229–1235, 1977

Arango V, Ernsberger P, Marzuk P, et al: Autoradiographic demonstration of increased serotonin 5-HT$_2$ and beta-adrenergic receptor binding sites in the brain of suicide victims. Arch Gen Psychiatry 47:1038–1047, 1990

Arato M, Frecska E, Tekes K, et al: Serotonergic interhemispheric asymmetry: gender differences in the orbital cortex. Acta Psychiatr Scand 84:110–111, 1991

Åsberg M, Träskman L, Thorén P: 5-HIAA in the cerebrospinal fluid: a biochemical suicide predictor? Arch Gen Psychiatry 33:1193–1197, 1976

Barratt ES, Patton JH: Impulsivity: cognitive, behavioral and psychophysiological correlates, in Biological Basis of Sensation-Seeking, Impulsivity and Anxiety. Edited by Zuckerman M. Hillsdale, NJ, Lawrence Erlbaum, 1983, pp 77–116

Brown CS, Kent TA, Bryant SG, et al: Blood platelet uptake of serotonin in episodic aggression. Psychiatry Res 27:5–12, 1989

Brown GL, Ebert MH, Goyer PF, et al: Aggression, suicide, and serotonin: relationship to CSF amine metabolites. Am J Psychiatry 139:741–746, 1982

Buss AH, Durkee A: An inventory for assessing different kinds of hostility. Journal of Consulting Psychology 21:343–349, 1957

Carlsson M, Carlsson A: A regional study of sex differences in rat brain serotonin. Prog Neuropsychopharmacol Biol Psychiatry 12:53–61, 1988

Charney DS, Goodman WK, Price LH, et al: Serotonin function in obsessive-compulsive disorder. Arch Gen Psychiatry 45:177–185, 1988

Coccaro EF, Siever LJ, Klar HM, et al: Serotonergic studies in patients with affective and personality disorders: correlates with suicidal and impulsive aggressive behavior. Arch Gen Psychiatry 46:587–599, 1989

Coccaro EF, Gabriel S, Siever LJ: Buspirone challenge: preliminary evidence for a role for central 5-HT$_{1A}$ receptor function in impulsive aggressive behavior in humans. Psychopharmacol Bull 26:393–405, 1990a

Coccaro EF, Siever LJ, Owen KR, et al: Serotonin in mood and personality disorders, in Serotonin in Major Psychiatric Disorders. Edited by Coccaro EF, Murphy D. Washington, DC, American Psychiatric Press, 1990b, pp 71–97

Coccaro EF, Silverman JM, Klar HM, et al: Familial correlates of reduced central serotonergic system function in patients with personality disorder. Arch Gen Psychiatry 51:318–324, 1994

Cooper JR, Bloom FE, Roth RH: The Biochemical Basis of Neuropharmacology, 6th Edition. New York, Oxford University Press, 1991

Dietz PE: Patterns of human violence, in Psychiatry Update: American Psychiatric Association Annual Review, Vol 6. Edited by Hales RE, Francis AJ. Washington, DC, American Psychiatric Press, 1987, pp 435–490

Hamilton M: A rating scale for depression. J Neurol Neurosurg Psychiatry 23:56–62, 1960

Heinsbroek RP, van Haaren F, Feenstra MG, et al: Sex differences in the effects of inescapable footshock on central catecholaminergic and serotonergic activity. Pharmacol Biochem Behav 37:539–550, 1990

Ieni JR, Tobach E, Zukin SR, et al: Multiple ^{3}H-imipramine binding sites in brains of male and female Frawn-Hooded and Long-Evan rats. Eur J Pharmacol 112:261–264, 1985

Jones JS, Stanley B, Mann J, et al: CSF 5-HIAA and HVA concentrations in elderly depressed patients who attempted suicide. Am J Psychiatry 147:1225–1227, 1990

Kellermann AL, Mercy JA: Men, women and violence: gender-specific differences in rates of fatal violence and victimization. J Trauma 33:1–5, 1992

Kostowski W, Valzelli L, Kozak W, et al: Activity of desipramine, fluoxetine and nomifensine on spontaneous and p-CPA-induced muricidal aggression. Pharmacological Research Communications 16:265–271, 1984

Kruesi MJ, Rapoport JL, Hamburger S, et al: Cerebrospinal fluid monoamine metabolites, aggression, and impulsivity in disruptive behavior disorders of children and adolescents. Arch Gen Psychiatry 47:419–426, 1990

Lepage P, Steiner M: Gender and serotonergic dysregulation: implications for late luteal phase dysphoric disorder, in Serotonin-Related Psychiatric Syndromes: Clinical and Therapeutic Links. Edited by Cassano GB, Akiskal HS. London, England, Royal Society of Medicine Services Limited, 1991, pp 131–142

Lidberg L, Åsberg M, Sunquist-Stensman M, et al: 5-hydroxyindoleacetic acid levels in attempted suicides who have killed their children (letter). Lancet 2:928, 1984

Lidberg L, Tuck JR, Åsberg M, et al: Homicide, suicide and CSF 5-HIAA. Acta Psychiatr Scand 71:230–236, 1985

Linnoila M, Virkkunen M, Scheinin M, et al: Low cerebrospinal fluid 5-hydroxyindoleacetic acid concentration differentiates impulsive from nonimpulsive violent behavior. Life Sci 33:2609–2614, 1983

Mann JJ, Arango V: Integration of neurobiology and psychopathology in a unified model of suicidal behavior. J Clin Psychopharmacol 12 (2, suppl):2S–7S, 1992

Marazziti D, Leo D, Conti L: Further evidence supporting the role of the serotonin system in suicidal behavior: a preliminary study of suicide attempters. Acta Psychiatr Scand 80:322–324, 1989

Meltzer HY, Arora RC: Platelet markers of suicidality. Ann N Y Acad Sci 487:271–280, 1986

Modai I, Apter A, Meltzer H, et al: Serotonin uptake by platelets of suicidal and aggressive adolescent psychiatric inpatients. Neuropsychobiology 21:9–13, 1989

Molina V, Ciesielski L, Gobaille S, et al: Inhibition of mouse killing behavior by serotonin-mimetic drugs: effects of partial alterations on serotonin transmission. Pharmacol Biochem Behav 27:123–131, 1987

Norden MJ: Fluoxetine in borderline personality disorder. Prog Neuropsychopharmacol Biol Psychiatry 13:885–893, 1989

O'Connor LH, Feder HH: Estradiol and progesterone influence L-5-hydroxytryptophan-induced myoclonus in male guinea pigs: sex differences in serotonin-steroid interactions. Brain Res 330:121–125, 1985

Pandey GN, Pandey SC, Janicak PG, et al: Platelet serotonin-2 receptor binding sites in depression and suicide. Biol Psychiatry 28:215–222, 1990

Ratey J, Sovner R, Parks A, et al: Buspirone treatment of aggression and anxiety in mentally retarded patients: a multiple-baseline, placebo, lead-in study. J Clin Psychiatry 52:159–162, 1991

Roy A, DeJong J, Linnoila M: Cerebrospinal fluid monoamine metabolites and suicidal behavior in depressed patients: a 5-year follow-up study. Arch Gen Psychiatry 46:609–612, 1989

Sheard MH, Marini JL, Bridges CI, et al: The effect of lithium on impulsive aggressive behavior in man. Am J Psychiatry 133:1409–1413, 1976

Siever LJ, Davis KL: A psychobiological perspective on the personality disorders. Am J Psychiatry 148:1647–1658, 1991

Siever LJ, Kahn RS, Lawlor BA, et al: Critical issues in defining the role of serotonin in psychiatric disorders. Pharmacol Rev 43:509–525, 1991

Siever LJ, Coccaro EF, Trestman RL, et al: The growth hormone response to clonidine in acute and remitted depressed male patients. Neuropsychopharmacology 6:165–177, 1992

Stark P, Fuller RW, Wong DT: The pharmacologic profile of fluoxetine. J Clin Psychiatry 46:7–13, 1985

Trestman RL, Coccaro EF, Mitropoulou V, et al: Differential biology of impulsivity, suicide and depression in personality disorders. Proceedings of the 23rd Congress of the International Society of Psychoneuroendocrinology, 1992a, p. 92

Trestman RL, Coccaro EF, Temple J, et al: Impulsivity and serotonin in borderline personality disorder. Paper presented at the 145th annual meeting of the American Psychiatric Association, Washington, DC, May 1992b

Vaillant GE, Perry JC: Personality disorders, in Comprehensive Textbook of Psychiatry/IV, 4th Edition. Edited by Kaplan HI, Sadock BJ. Baltimore, MD, Williams & Wilkins, 1985, p. 979

Valzelli L, Bernasconi S, Garattini S: p-chlorophenylalanine-induced muricidal aggression in male and female laboratory rats. Neuropsychobiology 7:315–320, 1981

Virkkunen M, Nuutila A, Goodwin FK, et al: Cerebrospinal fluid monoamine metabolite levels in male arsonists. Arch Gen Psychiatry 44:241–247, 1987

Yudofsky SC, Williams D, Gorman J: Propranolol in the treatment of rage and violent behavior in patients with chronic brain syndromes. Am J Psychiatry 138:218–220, 1981

Chapter 3

The Cholinergic and Noradrenergic Neurotransmitter Systems and Affective Instability in Borderline Personality Disorder

Bonnie Jean Steinberg, M.D.
Robert L. Trestman, M.D., Ph.D.
Larry J. Siever, M.D.

Affective instability, a central characteristic of borderline personality disorder (BPD), is defined in DSM-III-R (American Psychiatric Association 1987) as "marked shifts from baseline mood to depression, irritability, or anxiety, usually lasting a few hours and only rarely more than a few days" (p. 347). These unstable, rapidly changing moods are in contrast to what is found in classic mood disorders, which are characterized by a sustained, marked shift of affective state to either depression or elation. In BPD, affective shifts are sensitive to meaningful environmental events—such as separation, frustration of expectations, or criticism—that would induce a more modest response in other people. In addition, patients with BPD have poor impulse control, and their affective responses to frustration or disappointment may lead either to self-destructive or self-defeating behavior or to struggling with a significant other in an attempt to prevent abandonment. Instability of mood may interfere with an individual's capacity to develop stable representations of self and others and may result in difficulty developing or maintaining self-esteem.

A dimensional model of the Axis II disorders may be useful in understanding the psychobiology of BPD, and, more specifically, the trait of affective instability (Siever and Davis 1991). This dimensional model evolves from what is known currently about the biology of both Axis I and Axis II disorders and provides a theoretical framework for investigating biological hypotheses of Axis II disorders. Four major classes of Axis I disorders are the schizophrenic disorders, the mood disorders, the impulse control disorders, and the anxiety disorders. These classes correspond to disturbances in the functioning of the dimensions of 1) cognitive/perceptual organization, 2) affect regulation, 3) impulse control, and 4) anxiety modulation. These dimensions may have biological correlates. Although severe abnormalities associated with these dimensions may lead to Axis I disorders, biological correlates of these dimensions may also contribute to the maladaptive traits or behavioral predispositions that make up the personality disorders (Siever and Davis 1991).

This hypothesis can be understood more clearly by very briefly examining the relationship between schizophrenia and schizotypal personality disorder (SPD). Similar biological abnormalities are found in patients across the spectrum of schizophrenia-related disorders. For example, schizophrenic patients with cognitive and perceptual abnormalities display impairment of visual and auditory attention, such as smooth pursuit eye tracking abnormalities; these abnormalities have been found to correlate with deficit symptoms (Holzman et al. 1984). These abnormalities can also be found in patients with other schizophrenic spectrum disorders such as SPD (Siever et al. 1984). In addition, studies of dopaminergic function demonstrate a correlation both with the positive symptoms of schizophrenia and with the psychotic-like symptoms of schizotypal patients. Thus, disturbances in cognitive and perceptual organization, which can be found to a mild degree in SPD, are correlated with biological abnormalities related to the abnormalities on Axis I of schizophrenia.

As has been elaborated in Chapter 2, impulse control disorders appear to be related to a decrease in serotonergic function (Coccaro et al. 1989). Very briefly summarized, we find that Axis II dramatic cluster personality disorder patients are often impulsive. For example, people with BPD may make suicide attempts, have angry outbursts, get into fights, and abuse substances. These impulsive behaviors often appear to be in response to a disappointment or frustration in an important relationship. In antisocial personality disorder, impulsivity is manifest as stealing or lying. The trait of impulsivity may also contribute to the exaggerated displays of emotion in response to frustration seen in histrionic patients, or to the rage in response to criticism seen in narcissistic patients. In personality disorder patients with impulsive aggression, decreases in cerebrospinal fluid (CSF) 5-hydroxyindoleacetic acid (5-HIAA) and decreased prolactin response to fenfluramine have been demonstrated; these findings imply a relationship of impulsive aggression to serotonin.

In a similar vein, the mood disorders of Axis I may be related to the trait of affective instability. In patients with this trait, mood changes are marked and can last from minutes to hours and, rarely, for days. In contrast, in the major mood disorders, changes in mood last, by definition, for a minimum of 2 weeks. It has been hypothesized that depression may be a consequence, in part, of a relative excess of cholinergic activity, and that mania may result from a predominance of the adrenergic system (Janowsky et al. 1972a). It may be that these neurotransmitter systems contribute differentially to the trait of affective instability. For example, supersensitivity of the cholinergic system may contribute to a predisposition to dysphoria, and the noradrenergic system may contribute to an increased sensitivity to environmental events.

In affectively unstable individuals, rapid mood shifts are often seen in response to environmental stimuli, and perhaps a hyperreactivity to the environment may contribute to the exquisite rejection sensitivity that is characteristic of several of the personality disorders. Rejection sensitivity, at least in clinical work, appears to be a central theme among borderline patients. Patients with other personality disorders—in particular, those with histrionic, narcissistic, avoidant, and dependent personality disorders—also have symptoms that reflect excessive affective reactivity. When this trait of increased reactivity to the environment is combined with impulsivity, as in an individual with

BPD, the mixture may contribute to characteristically dysfunctional behaviors or actions. For example, anger in response to a rejection or disappointment may, in these patients, lead to various forms of impulsive, self-destructive threats or behavior, as is described in criterion 5 of DSM-III-R; "spending, sex, substance use, shoplifting, reckless driving, binge eating" (criterion 2); inappropriate displays of temper (criterion 4); or "frantic efforts to avoid real or imagined abandonment" (criterion 8) (American Psychiatric Association 1987). Emotional responses may be exaggerated in an attempt to influence the reactions of others in the environment and thereby help the borderline patient to modulate his or her own mood and self-perception. In Axis II anxious cluster patients, affective instability combined with anxiety/inhibition could contribute to dependent or avoidant personality characteristics. For example, an affectively reactive individual who is easily disappointed by separation or rejection might constantly anticipate separation or disappointment, and this outlook may lead to either avoidant or dependent patterns of behavior.

Thus far, however, there is no clear biological correlate to the affective instability/sensitivity of the personality disorders. State-dependent correlates of depression such as blunted thyroid-stimulating hormone response to thyroid-releasing hormone and escape of plasma cortisol from suppression by dexamethasone are not consistently abnormal in affectively unstable patients (Doerr and Berger 1983; Korzekwa et al. 1993). However, affective instability is a long-standing trait associated with personality disorders, which by definition incorporate enduring patterns of behavior. This is in contrast to the episodic major mood disorders. Affective instability is thus most likely correlated with a state-independent or trait biological abnormality. A logical starting point of investigation would be to explore the state-independent correlates of the major affective disorders.

There is a large body of work implicating the cholinergic and noradrenergic systems in the pathophysiology of the mood disorders. Increased responsiveness to the cholinergic system (or to the central neurotransmitter acetylcholine) is found in major depression (Janowsky and Risch 1987). Acetylcholinesterase inhibitors and muscarinic agonists, both of which increase cholinergic availability in the brain, create a depression-like syndrome in both animals (Janowsky et al. 1972a, 1972b) and humans (Davis et al. 1978; Janowsky et al. 1974). In both acutely depressed and remitted depressed patients, there is a decrease in rapid eye movement (REM) sleep latency (Sitaram et al. 1982), and this decrease can be enhanced by agents that increase central nervous system (CNS) cholinergic availability (Jones et al. 1985; Sitaram et al. 1982). Borderline patients also show decreased REM latency (Akiskal et al. 1985; McNamara et al. 1984), and enhancement of this REM latency with muscarinic agonists has been demonstrated in preliminary studies with borderline patients (Bell et al. 1983). Preliminary studies from our laboratory, as will be discussed below, also show that personality disorder patients with the trait of affective instability have a differential depressive-like response to physostigmine, an acetylcholinesterase inhibitor. These findings thus suggest that the cholinergic system may contribute to affective instability in personality disorder patients.

The noradrenergic system in part regulates engagement of the organism with the environment (Siever 1987). In major depression, interaction with the environment is decreased; this decreased interaction may lead to symptoms such as psychomotor retardation, withdrawal, and decreased concentration, corresponding to a hyporesponsive noradrenergic system (Siever and Davis 1985). In addition, a side effect of the lipophilic beta-blockers is the induction of depression (Roy et al. 1988). The noradrenergic system tends to be hyperactive in risk takers such as gamblers (Roy et al. 1988), and healthy individuals in certain circumstances become more irritable in response to agents that increase noradrenergic transmission in the CNS (Coccaro et al. 1991). Individuals with hysteroid dysphoria, who are characterized by increased emotional responsiveness, especially to rejection, may respond best to treatment with monoamine oxidase inhibitors (MAOIs), which increase noradrenergic availability (Gardner and Cowdry 1986). Increased reactivity to environmental events is characteristic of affective instability. It is then possible that a hyperresponsive noradrenergic system may also contribute to affective instability in personality disorder patients.

In this chapter we explore the relationship between the cholinergic and noradrenergic neurotransmitter systems and affective instability in borderline and other personality disorder patients.

THE CHOLINERGIC SYSTEM

The Cholinergic System in Mood Disorders

Acetylcholine is a neurotransmitter with many functions. It has effects on learning, memory, attention, mood, nociception, emotion, aggression, social play, exploration, grooming, odor aversion, sexual behavior, response to stress, thermoregulation, motor function, sleep, water intake, and neuroendocrine function (Bartus et al. 1987; Watson et al. 1987). In addition, as stated previously, increased cholinergic sensitivity has been linked to depression.

Several techniques are used to increase cholinergic availability in the CNS. Use of these techniques allows us either to mimic the effects of increased acetylcholine on or to test the sensitivity to acetylcholine of that system. One technique is to block acetylcholinesterase, the enzyme that breaks down acetylcholine. Examples of agents that block acetylcholinesterase include physostigmine and diisopropylfluorophosphate (DFP). Another technique involves the direct stimulation of muscarinic acetylcholine receptors with agonists such as arecoline, oxotremorine, and RS86. An alternate technique is to block the muscarinic receptors and thus inhibit the function of acetylcholine. Muscarinic antagonists such as atropine and scopolamine can be used in this manner (Table 3–1).

Several preclinical animal models of depression and the cholinergic system have been developed. Cholinomimetics administered to a number of animal species produce behavioral inhibitory effects that include lethargy, hypoactivity, and decrease in self-stimulation, all of which may be considered as animal models of depression (Janowsky et al. 1972a, 1972b). Normal rats whose muscarinic receptors have been upregulated (i.e., increased) as the result of withdrawal of chronic scopolamine treatment show a greater degree of immobility in the forced swim test (a behavioral model of depression) (Overstreet et al.

Table 3–1. Neuroendocrine challenges to the cholinergic system

Cholinergic availability	
Increased	**Decreased**
Cholinesterase inhibitors	Acetylcholinesterase
Physostigmine	
Diisopropylfluorophosphate (DFP)	
Muscarinic acetylcholine receptor agonists	Muscarinic acetylcholine receptor antagonists
Arecoline	Atropine
Oxotremorine	Scopolamine
RS86	

1986), whereas anticholinergic drugs reduce behavioral immobility in the forced swim test (Janowsky and Risch 1987).

Two strains of rats have been developed and bred for their cholinergic supersensitivity. One is the Flinders Sensitive Line (Overstreet et al. 1988), which exhibits increased sensitivity to muscarinic agonists and cholinomimetics. These rats have elevated numbers of hippocampal and striatal muscarinic acetylcholine receptors and decreased body weight and locomotor activity. They demonstrate less activity and increased sensitivity in response to the induction of behavioral immobility following a forced swim test (Overstreet 1986; Overstreet and Russell 1982, 1984; Overstreet et al. 1988), and also exhibit enhanced responsiveness to stimuli that elicit affective aggression (Pucilowski et al. 1990–1991). A second strain of rats, the Roman Low Avoiding Strain (Bignami 1965; Martin et al. 1981), which has high levels of choline acetyltransferase activity in the striatum and hippocampus, demonstrates less ability to learn an active avoidance response and is more sensitive to the behavioral effects of oxotremorine and physostigmine (Martin et al. 1981).

In humans there is a large body of evidence that dysregulation of the cholinergic system is implicated, at least in part, in the major mood disorders. Centrally acting cholinomimetics lead to a depressive-like syndrome in a variety of patient groups, and mood disorder patients are more sensitive to physostigmine infusion than are nonpsychiatrically ill control subjects (Janowsky et al. 1974). Studies in manic and hypomanic bipolar patients have found an increase in depressive symptoms with physostigmine infusion (Davis et al. 1978; Janowsky et al. 1973). The same effect was seen in unipolar depressed and schizoaffective depressed patients (Janowsky et al. 1972b), in euthymic bipolar patients on lithium, and in euthymic depressed patients (Oppenheim et al. 1979). Arecoline, a cholinergic agonist, can cause increased depression, hostility, and anxiety in depressed patients (Risch et al. 1983).

Cholinomimetics also cause sleep changes that are characteristic of depression, such as decreased REM latency and increased REM density (Gillin et al. 1991); these REM sleep changes are again more pronounced in depressed patients (Gillin et al. 1991; Sitaram et al. 1982) and bipolar patients (Nurnberger et al. 1989). This increased responsiveness to cholinomimetics suggests increased sensitivity to acetylcholine in depressed patients. Most studies show increased responsivity to cholinomimetics to be state independent, or a trait correlate of mood disorders, although one recent study of asymptomatic patients who had been medication free for an average of 3 years found no change in REM sleep in response to the cholinergic agonist RS86 (Riemann and Berger 1989). RS86, however, may not stimulate the release of cortisol and therefore may constitute an inadequate challenge (Berger et al. 1991).

Cholinomimetics typically produce changes in the hypothalamic-pituitary-adrenal (HPA) axis that are similar to those seen in depression—namely, elevation of serum adrenocorticotropic hormone (ACTH), cortisol, and β-endorphin. These changes in the HPA axis in response to cholinomimetics are usually greater in affective disorder patients than in control subjects (Risch et al. 1983). Infusion with pyridostigmine, an indirect cholinergic agent thought to release growth hormone by decreasing inhibitory somatostatin tone, stimulated a greater growth hormone response in depressed patients than in control subjects (O'Keane et al. 1992); this study provides further evidence for cholinergic supersensitivity in depression. Thus, REM sleep, mediated in part by the cholinergic system, is dysregulated in depressed patients, and this decrease in REM latency can be exacerbated by cholinomimetics.

The Cholinergic System and Affective Instability

A number of studies have examined the cholinergic system in healthy individuals. These studies have found that cholinomimetics, both muscarinic agonists and cholinesterase inhibitors, can produce a depression-like response when administered to healthy control subjects (Doerr and Berger 1983; Modestin et al. 1973; Risch et al. 1981). This response appears to be dose dependent (Fritze et al. 1988). In a study of healthy men, behavioral and cardiovascular response to physostigmine correlated with patterns of behavior often associated with depression—that is, depressive attitudes and passive, helpless strategies for coping with stress. Response to physostigmine was also correlated with trait (long-standing) irritability and emotional lability. The metabolic and neuroendocrine responses to physostigmine infusion, however, were not correlated with personality (Fritze et al. 1990). In healthy men without a personal or family history of depression, physostigmine infusion resulted in behavioral inhibitory changes, namely anergia, lethargy, decreased spontaneous activity, and diminished verbal fluency. These inhibitory changes occurred without dysphoric changes in mood or changes in attention/cognition (Silva et al. 1992). Taken together as a group, these studies suggest that behavioral inhibition, emotional lethargy, and slowed thinking in personality disorders are affected by the cholinergic system, but that a biological vulnerability to depression may be necessary for concomitant changes in mood and attention.

Further data for mediation by the cholinergic system of both affective instability and its biological correlates come from studies of patients with BPD. Borderline patients show decreased and more variable REM latency without a neuroendocrine challenge (Akiskal et al. 1985; Bell et al. 1983; McNamara et al. 1984) and enhanced reduction in REM latency in response to cholinomimetics (Bell et al. 1983). Reduction in REM latency in response to physostigmine is also seen to some degree in nonpsychiatrically ill control subjects (Risch et al. 1983).

Cholinomimetic (Physostigmine) Challenge in Personality Disorder Patients With Affective Instability

In a study in our laboratory, the mood response to physostigmine was evaluated in personality disorder patients. Eight patients were assessed at baseline with the Schedule for Affective Disorders and Schizophrenia (SADS; Endicott and Spitzer 1978), the Structured Interview for DSM-III Personality Disorders (SIDP; Stangl et al. 1985), and the Affective Lability Scale (ALS; Harvey et al. 1989). There were six personality disorder patients who met the criterion of affective instability as defined in the DSM-III-R criteria for BPD and two patients who did not meet this affective lability criterion but who did meet criteria for a personality disorder diagnosis. Five of the patients met criteria for BPD; four met criteria for other personality disorders. (Some subjects met criteria for more than one personality disorder). None of the patients had concurrent major depression, but approximately half of the patients had a history of one or more episodes of major depression.

Following an overnight fast, patients were catheterized intravenously and given glycopyrrolate to counter the peripheral effects of physostigmine. Patients were given two infusions administered 2 days apart. Each infusion was at the same time of the day, 10 A.M, and each was performed under double-blind conditions. One infusion was physostigmine, 14 µg/kg in a 10cc normal saline iv that was infused over a period of 10 minutes. The other infusion was 10cc normal saline as a placebo control. Vital signs and electrocardiograms (ECGs) were monitored, and the patients were observed throughout the procedure.

At −60 minutes, + 20 minutes, and + 75 minutes, patients were administered the Profile of Mood States (POMS; Lorr et al. 1971) and a 100mm mood line visual analog scale. The subjects who met the criterion for affective instability had a placebo-corrected peak POMS depression subscale response to physostigmine of 9.8 ± 3.4, compared with 2.5 ± 3.5 for those who did not meet the criterion for affective instability ($t = 2.57$, df = 6, $P < .05$) (Steinberg et al. 1993).

Although the sample size is small, these data suggest that patients with the trait of affective instability are more sensitive to cholinergic activity and that they respond to an increase in cholinergic availability with a shift in mood toward depression. This response strongly implies that the trait of affective instability has a biological correlate, at least in part, in increased sensitivity of the cholinergic system.

THE NORADRENERGIC SYSTEM

Studies of Arousal and Engagement With the Environment

The noradrenergic system modulates arousal and engagement with the environment. In primates, the locus coeruleus, the primary noradrenergic nucleus of the brain, has decreased firing during vegetative activities such as eating, sleeping, and grooming (Aston-Jones and Bloom 1981). This decreased activation also occurs during withdrawal from the environment in response to separation (McKinney et al. 1984). When organisms are presented with novel or threatening stimuli, the activity in the locus coeruleus is increased (Aston-Jones and Bloom 1981; Levine et al. 1990). Noradrenergic activity is also associated with irritable, aggressive, or defensive behavior (Levine et al. 1990). In mice, administration of tyrosine, a norepinephrine precursor, leads to increased territorial aggression (Thurmond et al. 1977). Shock-induced stress in rats leads to an increase in synthesis of norepinephrine and an increase in irritable aggression (Lamprecht et al. 1972; Stolk et al. 1974). Administration of an alpha$_2$-noradrenergic antagonist to rats leads to an increase in noradrenergic activity as well as to an increase in rough-and-tumble play (Siviy et al. 1990). Thus, decreased noradrenergic activity is associated with withdrawal from the environment and increased noradrenergic activity is associated with heightened engagement with, and reactivity to, the environment.

The Noradrenergic System in Mood Disorders

Major depression is associated with a hyporesponsive noradrenergic system. This hyporesponsivity has been demonstrated in studies that show a decreased production of the metabolites of norepinephrine in depressed patients. These metabolites include vanillylmandelic acid (VMA) and normetanephrine (Koslow et al. 1983). In some depressed patients, there is a decrease in CSF 3-methoxy-4-hydroxyphenylglycol (MHPG) (Post et al. 1984), also a metabolite of norepinephrine. Alpha$_2$-adrenergic receptor function has been shown to be decreased in patients with major depression in studies that reveal a decreased growth hormone (GH) response to the alpha$_2$-adrenergic agonist clonidine (Ansseau et al. 1984; Charney et al. 1982; Siever et al. 1982). This blunted GH response is not present in reactive depression (Checkley et al. 1981, 1984; Matussek et al. 1980), serious medical illness (Lechin et al. 1985), or schizophrenia (Lal et al. 1975; Matussek et al. 1980), although it can be found in patients with anxiety disorders such as obsessive-compulsive disorder (Siever et al. 1983) and panic disorder with agoraphobia (Siever et al. 1985).

The Noradrenergic System and Engagement With the Environment

The noradrenergic system is hyperresponsive in individuals with high levels of engagement with the environment. Pathological gamblers, for example, have increased measures of arousal (Eysenck 1967), susceptibility to boredom, and sensation seeking (Dickerson et al. 1987). People with increased sensation-seeking behavior demonstrate elevated concentrations of CSF MHPG and greater outputs of norepinephrine (Roy et al. 1988). CSF MHPG, plasma MHPG and urinary VMA, and the sum of all urinary outputs of norepinephrine and its metabolites are correlated with extroversion, a dimension that is theoretically related to arousal (Eysenck 1967). In addition, increased GH response to clonidine is found in children with attention-deficit hyperactivity disorder (ADHD) compared with healthy control subjects; this GH response is decreased in ADHD patients treated with methylphenidate (Hunt et al. 1984). Thus, in people with high reactivity to and engagement with the environment, increased noradrenergic function has been found.

Studies Relating to Affective Instability

Studies With Healthy Volunteers and BPD Patients

We have found, in a study of patients and normal volunteers, that GH responses to clonidine were significantly correlated with the Buss-Durkee Hostility Inventory (BDHI; Buss and Durkee 1957). Irritability subscale scores correlated with GH response more strongly in both healthy control subjects and personality disorder patients than in patients with major depression (Coccaro et al. 1991). The personality characteristic of behavioral irritability may be related to central adrenergic hyperresponsiveness in control subjects and personality disorder patients. DSM-III hysteroid dysphoria patients, most of whom met criteria for BPD (Liebowitz and Klein 1981), have been characterized as displaying increased emotional reactivity to the environment, especially to loss. These patients have been found to be responsive to pharmacological treatment with the MAOIs—pharmacological agents that are believed to stabilize the function of the noradrenergic system. Affective instability in some personality disorder patients has been shown in some studies to respond to lithium carbonate (Rifkin et al. 1972) and to carbamazepine (Gardner and Cowdry 1986), both of which stabilize neurotransmitter function (although not exclusively catecholaminergic function).

The Noradrenergic System and Affective Instability

Studies to Date

We recently studied a larger cohort of patients in a protocol similar to that described above. Thirty-one patients with DSM-III personality disorders, 19 males and 12 females, were studied in order to better appreciate the relationship between noradrenergic function and irritability and hostility. Patients were diagnosed with the SADS, the SIDP-R, the BDHI, and the Barratt Impulsivity Scale (BIS; Barratt and Patton 1983). No patient had a history of mania, schizophrenia, schizoaffective disorder, or unspecified psychosis.

Following an overnight fast and bed rest, patients received an intravenous catheter that was then maintained with normal saline. Lumbar puncture was performed between 9 and 10 A.M. by a qualified physician. CSF samples were used to measure CSF MHPG. Simultaneous plasma MHPG levels were drawn. On a separate day, again following an overnight fast and bedrest, an intravenous catheter was placed in patient subjects and the intravenous line maintained with normal saline infusion. Plasma norepinephrine, MHPG, and GH levels were drawn at 9:30, 9:45, and 10:00 A.M. Patients were then given 2 μg/kg of clonidine in 10 cc of normal saline that was infused intravenously over 5 minutes. Plasma GH concentrations were drawn at 30-minute intervals for 3 hours.

Male patients with BPD had increased 60-minute (peak) GH response to clonidine (13.8 ng/ml versus 6.8 ng/ml at 60 minutes; $n = 3$ BPD, 16 non-BPD) and increased basal CSF MHPG (26.5 ng/ml versus 13.9 ng/ml; $n = 4$ BPD, 10 non-BPD) when compared with male non-BPD patients. This difference was statistically significant when criteria for the diagnosis of BPD were relaxed to four criteria (rather than five). In personality disorder patients, basal plasma norepinephrine correlated positively with risk taking and impulsivity (all subjects: BIS risk-taking subscale $r = .48, n = 29, P < .004$; BIS total $r = .32, n = 29, P < .05$; males: BIS risk-taking subscale $r = .52, n = 18, P < .012$; BIS total $r = .037, n = 18, P < .07$; females: BIS risk-taking subscale $r = .059, n = 11, P < .06$). In the sample of personality disorder patients, GH response to clonidine infusion correlated positively with measures of irritability (BDHI irritability subscale $r = .26, P < .1$) and verbal hostility (BDHI verbal hostility subscale $r = .36, P < .05$) (BDHI total $r = .23, P < .1$) (Trestman et al. 1992).

Thus, BPD is correlated with increased responsiveness of the noradrenergic system. Personality disorder patients with high levels of risk taking, irritability, and verbal aggression, all of which are influenced by engagement with the environment, appear to have hyperresponsive noradrenergic systems. These data suggest that increased responsiveness of the noradrenergic system is correlated with increased reactivity and sensitivity to the environment.

SUMMARY AND CONCLUSIONS

Affective instability, a trait central to BPD but also found in other personality disorders, is characterized by marked shifts in mood, irritability, or anxiety that usually last hours and, rarely, days. There may be two interactive components that contribute to affective instability: one a dysphoric, or mood, component and the other an excessive reactivity to the environment component. The cholinergic system may be primarily implicated in the affective instability component and the noradrenergic system implicated in the environmental hyperreactivity component.

An examination of the evidence for a role for the cholinergic system in personality disorder patients with affective instability reveals some promising findings. For example, we have demonstrated that physostigmine infusion in personality disorder patients who possess the trait of affective instability, as well as in patients with BPD per se, produced a differential depressive response that was statistically significant when compared with that of control groups. Although the sample size was small, these findings suggest that personality disorder patients with affective instability, including patients with BPD, appear to have a heightened sensitivity to acetylcholine.

There is some evidence implicating the noradrenergic system as also playing an important role in affective instability. We have shown that the increased responsiveness of the noradrenergic system in healthy control subjects and personality disorder patients is correlated with the trait characteristic of irritability. In an expanded cohort, personality disorder patients with increased irritability in general, and patients with BPD in particular, demonstrated indices that reflect increased activity of the noradrenergic system, both at baseline and after challenge with clonidine. Although this work is preliminary, these data suggest that personality disorder patients with high levels of environmental engagement have increased reactivity of the noradrenergic system. Engagement with the environment can be viewed as a major characteristic of the trait of affective instability. Catecholamine metabolism in BPD is explored in Chapter 4.

Affective reactivity may make it difficult to develop stable representations of self or others, thereby contributing significantly to the development of poor self-esteem. When this trait is combined with other maladaptive traits in a given individual, certain dysfunctional personality patterns may ensue. For example, patients with BPD may exhibit affective instability as well as impulsivity. In these patients, an affectively charged rejection or disappointment may lead to impulsive self-destructive or self-defeating behaviors. In individuals with anxiety or inhibition and affective instability, disappointments due to separation or rejection may lead to a constant anxious anticipation of separation or disappointment, which in turn may contribute to avoidant or dependent behavior.

The trait of affective instability, a central feature of BPD as well as of several other cluster B personality disorders, is characterized by rapid mood shifts, often in response to meaningful environmental events. An examination of the known biology of the Axis I mood disorders suggests a potential biological basis for the trait of affective instability. Indeed, there is some preliminary evidence that both the cholinergic system, by regulating mood, and also the noradrenergic system, by regulating engagement with the environment, contribute to this trait.

Although most of these data are preliminary, they suggest areas for future investigation. These areas include a more precise investigation of the functioning and regulation of the cholinergic and noradrenergic neurotransmitter systems in affective instability, as well as how each, individually and in concert, impacts on the specific functions described. Another fruitful area for further investigation would be the study of the interaction of this trait, affective instability, with other dimensions of psychobiology of the personality disorders, such as impulsivity. While investigation of these possible interactions seems most promising for cluster B personality disorder patients, a better understanding of the effects of affective instability on anxiety and inhibition of behavior as manifested in cluster C personality disorder patients, and on cognitive and perceptual organization as revealed particularly in cluster A personality disorder patients, could have an important impact on our appreciation and treatment of the entire range of patients with Axis II disorders.

REFERENCES

Akiskal HS, Yerevarian BI, Davis GC, et al: The nosologic status of borderline personality: clinical and polysomnographic study. Am J Psychiatry 142:192–198, 1985

American Psychiatric Association: Diagnostic and Statistical Manual of Mental Disorders, 3rd Edition, Revised. Washington, DC, American Psychiatric Association, 1987

Ansseau M, Schaeyvert M, Dumont A, et al: Concurrent use of REM latency, dexamethasone suppression, clonidine, and apomorphine tests as biological markers of endogenous depression: a pilot study. Psychiatry Res 12:261–272, 1984

Aston-Jones G, Bloom FE: Norepinephrine-containing locus coeruleus neurons in behaving rats exhibit pronounced responses to non-noxious environmental stimuli. J Neurosci 1:887–900, 1981

Barratt ES, Patton JH. Impulsivity: cognitive, behavioral and psychophysiological correlates, in Biological Basis of Sensation-Seeking, Impulsivity and Anxiety. Edited by Zuckerman M. Hillsdale, NJ, Lawrence Erlbaum, 1983, pp 77–116

Bartus RT, Dean RL, Flicker C: Cholinergic psychopharmacology: an integration of human and animal research on memory, in Psychopharmacology: The Third Generation of Progress. Edited by Meltzer HY. New York, Raven, 1987, pp 219–233

Bell J, Grummet M, Lycaki H, et al: The effect of borderline personality disorder on sleep EEG state and trait markers of depression, in Abstracts of the 38th Meeting of the Society of Biological Psychiatry, May 1983

Berger M, Riemann D, Krieg C: Cholinergic drugs as diagnostic and therapeutic tools in affective disorders. Acta Psychiatr Scand/Suppl 366:52–60, 1991

Bignami G: Selection for high rates and low rates of avoidance conditioning in the rat. Animal Behavior 13:221–227, 1965

Buss AH, Durkee A: An inventory for assessing different kinds of hostility. Journal of Consulting Psychology 21:343–349, 1957

Charney DS, Heninger GA, Sternberg DE, et al: Adrenergic receptor sensitivity in depression: effects of clonidine in depressed and healthy subjects. Arch Gen Psychiatry 39:290–294, 1982

Checkley SA, Slade AP, Shur E: Growth hormone and other responses to clonidine in patients with endogenous depression. Br J Psychiatry 138:51–55, 1981

Checkley SA, Glass IB, Thompson C, et al: The GH response to clonidine in endogenous as compared with reactive depression. Psychol Med 14:773–77, 1984

Coccaro EF, Siever LJ, Klar HM, et al: Serotonergic studies in patients with affective and personality disorders: correlates with suicidal and impulsive aggressive behavior. Arch Gen Psychiatry 46:587–599, 1989 (correction, 47:124, 1990)

Coccaro EF, Lawrence T, Trestman RL, et al: Growth hormone responses to intravenous clonidine challenge correlate with behavioral irritability in psychiatric patients and in healthy volunteers. Psychiatry Res 39:129–139, 1991

Davis KL, Berger PA, Hollister LE, et al: Physostigmine in mania. Arch Gen Psychiatry 35:119–122, 1978

Dickerson M, Hinchy J, Falve J: Chasing, arousal and sensation seeking in off-course gamblers. Br J Addict 82:673–680, 1987

Doerr P, Berger M: Physostigmine-induced escape from dexamethasone suppression in normal adults. Biol Psychiatry 18:261–268, 1983

Endicott J, Spitzer RL: A diagnostic interview: the schedule for affective disorders and schizophrenia. Arch Gen Psychiatry 35:837–844, 1978

Eysenck H: The Biological Basis of Personality. Springfield, IL, Charles C Thomas, 1967

Fritze J, Sofic E, Riederer P, et al: Endocrine parameters and biogenic amines in relationship to psychopathology after cholinergic drug challenge (RS86). Psychiatry Res 25:339–348, 1988

Fritze J, Sofic E, Muller T, et al: Cholinergic-adrenergic balance, II: relationship between drug sensitivity and personality. Psychiatry Res 34:271–279, 1990

Gardner DL, Cowdry RW: Positive effects of carbamazepine on behavioral dyscontrol in borderline personality disorder. Am J Psychiatry 143:519–522, 1986

Gillin JC, Sutton L, Ruiz C, et al: The cholinergic rapid eye movement induction test with arecoline in depression. Arch Gen Psychiatry 48:264–270, 1991

Harvey PD, Greenberg BR, Serper MR: The affective lability scales: development, reliability and validity. J Clin Psychol 45:786–793, 1989

Holzman PS, Solomon CM, Levin S, et al: Pursuit eye movement dysfunctions in schizophrenia: family evidence for specificity. Arch Gen Psychiatry 41:136–139, 1984

Hunt RD, Cohen DJ, Anderson G, et al: Possible change in noradrenergic receptor sensitivity following methylphenidate treatment: growth hormone and MHPG response to clonidine challenge in children with attention deficit disorder and hyperactivity. Life Sci 35:885–897, 1984

Janowsky DS, Risch CS: Role of acetylcholine mechanisms in the affective disorders, in Psychopharmacology: The Third Generation of Progress. Edited by Meltzer HY. New York, Raven, 1987, pp 527–534

Janowsky DS, El-Yousef MK, Davis JM, et al: A cholinergic-adrenergic hypothesis of mania and depression. Lancet 2:632–635, 1972a

Janowsky DS, El-Yousef MK, Davis JM, et al: Cholinergic antagonism of methylphenidate-induced stereotyped behavior. Psychopharmacologia 27:295–314, 1972b

Janowsky DS, El-Yousef MK, Davis JM, et al: Parasympathetic suppression of manic symptoms by physostigmine. Arch Gen Psychiatry 28:542–547, 1973

Janowsky DS, El-Yousef MK, Davis JM: Acetylcholine and depression. Psychosom Med 36:248–257, 1974

Jones D, Kalwala S, Bell J, et al: Cholinergic REM induction response correlation with major depressive subtype. Psychiatry Res 14:99–110, 1985

Korzekwa M, Links P, Steiner M: Biological markers in borderline personality disorder: new perspectives. Can J Psychiatry 36 (suppl 1, Feb):1–5, 1993

Koslow SH, Maas JW, Bowden CL, et al: CSF and urinary biogenic amines and metabolites in depression and mania: a controlled univariate analysis. Arch Gen Psychiatry 40:999–1010, 1983

Lal S, Tolis G, Martin JB, et al: Effect of clonidine in growth hormone, prolactin, luteinizing hormone, follicle-stimulating hormone, and thyroid-stimulating hormone in the serum of normal men. J Clin Endocrinol Metab 41:827–832, 1975

Lamprecht F, Eichelman B, Thoa NB, et al: Rat fighting behavior: serum dopamine-B-hydroxylase and hypothalamic tyrosine hydroxylase. Science 177:1214–1215, 1972

Lechin F, van der Dijs B, Jakobowicz D, et al: Effects of clonidine on blood pressure, noradrenaline, cortisol, growth hormone, and prolactin plasma levels in high and low intestinal tone subjects. Neuroendocrinology 40:253–261, 1985

Levine ES, Litto WJ, Jacobs BL: Activity of cat locus coeruleus noradrenergic neurons during the defense reaction. Brain Res 531:189–195, 1990

Liebowitz MR, Klein DF: Interrelationship of hysteroid dysphoria and borderline personality disorder. Psychiatr Clin North Am 4:67–87, 1981

Lorr M, McNair DM, Droppleman LF: Manual: Profile of Mood States. San Diego, CA, Educational and Industrial Testing Service, 1971

Martin JR, Overstreet DH, Driscoll P, et al: Effects of scopolamine, pilocarpine, and oxotremorine on the exploratory behavior of two psychogenetically selected lines of rats in a complex maze. Psychopharmacology 72:135–142, 1981

Matussek N, Ackenheil M, Hippius H, et al: Effect of clonidine on growth hormone release in psychiatric patients and controls. Psychiatry Res 2:25–36, 1980

McKinney WT, Moran EC, Kraemer GW: Separation in nonhuman primates as a model for human depression: neurobiological implications, in Neurobiology of Mood Disorders. Edited by Post RM, Ballenger JC. Baltimore, MD, Williams & Wilkins, 1984, pp 393–406

McNamara E, Reynolds CF III, Soloff PH, et al: EEG sleep evaluation of depression in borderline patients. Am J Psychiatry 141:182–186, 1984

Modestin JJ, Schwartz RB, Hunger J: Zur Frage der Beeinflussung schizophrener Symptome dur Physostigmin. Pharmacopsychiatria 6:300–304, 1973

Nurnberger J Jr, Berrettini W, Mendelson W, et al: Measuring cholinergic sensitivity, I: arecoline effects in bipolar patients. Biol Psychiatry 25:610–617, 1989

O'Keane V, O'Flynn K, Lucey J, et al: Pyridostigmine-induced growth hormone responses in healthy and depressed subjects: evidence for cholinergic supersensitivity in depression. Psychol Med 22:55–60, 1992

Oppenheim G, Ebstein RP, Belmaker RH: Effect of lithium on the physostigmine induced behavioral syndrome and plasma cyclic GMP. J Psychiatr Res 15:133–138, 1979

Overstreet DH: Selective breeding for increased cholinergic function: development of a new animal model of depression. Biol Psychiatry 21:49–58, 1986

Overstreet DH, Russell RW: Selective breeding for diisopropyl fluorophosphate-sensitivity: behavioural effects of cholinergic agonists and antagonists. Psychopharmacology 78:150–154, 1982

Overstreet DH, Russell RW: Selective breeding for differences in cholinergic function: sex differences in the genetic regulation of sensitivity to the anticholinesterase DFP. Behav Neural Biol 40:227–238, 1984

Overstreet DH, Janowsky DS, Gillin JC, et al: Stress-induced immobility in rats with cholinergic supersensitivity. Biol Psychiatry 21:657–664, 1986

Overstreet DH, Russell RW, Crocker AD, et al: Genetic and pharmacological models of cholinergic supersensitivity and affective disorders. Experientia 44:465–472, 1988

Post RM, Jimerson DC, Ballenger JC, et al: Cerebrospinal fluid norepinephrine and its metabolites in manic-depressive illness, in Neurobiology of Mood Disorders. Edited by Post RM, Ballenger JC. Baltimore, MD, Williams & Wilkins, 1984, pp 539–553

Pucilowski O, Eichelman B, Overstreet DH, et al: Enhanced affective aggression in genetically bred hypercholinergic rats. Neuropsychobiology 24:37–41, 1990–1991

Riemann D, Berger M: EEG sleep in depression and in remission and the REM sleep response to the cholinergic agonist RS86. Neuropsychopharmacology 2:145–152, 1989

Rifkin A, Quitkin F, Carillo C, et al: Lithium carbonate in emotionally unstable character disorder. Arch Gen Psychiatry 27:519–523, 1972

Risch SC, Cohen PM, Janowsky KS, et al: Physostigmine induction of depressive symptomatology in normal human subjects. Psychiatry Res 4:89–94, 1981

Risch SC, Siever LJ, Gillin JC, et al: Differential mood effects of arecoline in depressed patients and normal volunteers. Psychopharmacol Bull 19:696–698, 1983

Roy A, Adinoff B, Linnoila M: Acting out hostility in normal volunteers: negative correlation with levels of 5-HIAA in cerebrospinal fluid. Psychiatry Res 24:187–194, 1988

Siever LJ: Role of noradrenergic mechanisms in the etiology of the affective disorders, in Psychopharmacology: The Third Generation of Progress. Edited by Meltzer HY. New York, Raven, 1987, pp 493–504

Siever LJ, Davis KL: Overview: towards a dysregulation hypothesis of depression. Am J Psychiatry 142:1017–1031, 1985

Siever LJ, Davis KL: A psychobiological perspective on the personality disorders. Am J Psychiatry 148:1647–1658, 1991

Siever LJ, Uhde TW, Silberman E, et al: The growth hormone response to clonidine as a probe of noradrenergic receptor responsiveness in affective disorder patients and controls. Psychiatry Res 6:171–183, 1982

Siever LJ, Insel TR, Jimerson DC, et al: Growth hormone response to clonidine in obsessive-compulsive patients. Br J Psychiatry 142:184–187, 1983

Siever LJ, Coursey RD, Alterman IS, et al: Impaired smooth pursuit eye movement: a vulnerability marker for schizotypal personality disorder in a normal volunteer population. Am J Psychiatry 141:1560–1566, 1984

Siever LJ, Uhde TW, Insel TR, et al: Biologic alterations in the primary affective disorders and other tricyclic-response disorders. Prog Neuropsychopharmacol Biol Psychiatry 9:15–24, 1985

Silva SG, Stern RA, Golder RN, et al: The effects of physostigmine on behavioral inhibition, cognition and mood in healthy males. Paper presented at the 42nd annual meeting of the Society of Biological Psychiatry, Washington, DC, May 1992

Sitaram N, Nurnberger J, Gershon ES, et al: Cholinergic regulation of mood and REM sleep: a potential model and marker for vulnerability to depression. Am J Psychiatry 139:571–576, 1982

Siviy SM, Atrens DM, Menendez JA: Idazoxan increases rough-and-tumble play, activity and exploration in juvenile rats. Psychopharmacology 100:119–123, 1990

Stangl D, Pfohl B, Zimmerman M, et al: A structured interview for the DSM-III personality disorders: preliminary report. Arch Gen Psychiatry 42:591–596, 1985

Steinberg B, Weston S, Trestman RL, et al: Affective instability in personality disordered patients correlates with mood response to physostigmine challenge. Abstracts of the 48th Meeting of the Society of Biological Psychiatry, May 1993 (Biol Psychiatry 33[6A]:86A [Abstract 180], 1993)

Stolk JM, Conner RL, Levine S, et al: Brain norepinephrine metabolism and shock-induced fighting behavior in rats: differential effects of shock and fighting on the neurochemical response to a common footshock stimulus. J Pharmacol Exp Ther 190:193–209, 1974

Thurmond JB, Lasley SM, Conkin AI, et al: Effects of dietary tyrosine, phenylalanine and tryptophan on aggression in mice. Pharmacol Biochem Behav 6:475–478, 1977

Trestman RL, Coccaro EF, Mitropoulou V, et al: Differential biology of impulsivity, suicide and depression in the personality disorders. Proceedings of the 23rd Congress of the International Society of Psychoneuroendocrinology, 1992, p 92

Watson M, Roeske WR, Yamamura HI: Cholinergic receptor heterogeneity, in Psychopharmacology: The Third Generation of Progress. Edited by Meltzer HY. New York, Raven, 1987, pp 241–248

Chapter 4

Peripheral Catecholamine Alterations in Borderline Personality Disorder

Rachel Yehuda, Ph.D.
Steven M. Southwick, M.D.
Bruce D. Perry, M.D., Ph.D.
Earl L. Giller, M.D., Ph.D

Considerable attention has been focused on the interface between borderline personality disorder (BPD) and major depressive disorder (MDD) (Gunderson and Elliott 1985; Gunderson and Phillips 1991). The elucidation of this relationship has important implications for our understanding and treatment of both disorders. Although several hypotheses have been raised concerning the relationship between these two syndromes, questions still remain about the core similarities between depressive phenomenology in borderline patients and major depression patients. In this chapter, we briefly review biological studies of BPD and explore the utility of indices of catecholamine metabolism in further elucidating the relationship between BPD and major depression. Our data consistently suggest that patients with BPD can be differentiated from those with MDD on at least two measures of catecholamine metabolism: platelet monoamine oxidase (MAO) activity and platelet alpha$_2$-adrenergic receptor binding. The biological alterations observed in BPD have pointed us in the direction of exploring the interface between BPD and anxiety disorders. As will be described in greater detail below, the biological changes that we have observed in BPD are similar to the changes we have observed in posttraumatic stress disorder

(PTSD). These results, which are compatible with those of recent studies that have conceptualized BPD as a type of traumatic stress response disorder related to chronic early abuse (Gunderson and Sabo 1993; Herman 1992; Herman et al. 1989; van der Kolk et al. 1991), underscore the importance of evaluating the relationship between BPD and anxiety disorders.

THE ASSOCIATION OF BORDERLINE PERSONALITY DISORDER AND MAJOR DEPRESSIVE DISORDER

Conceptual Framework of the Borderline–Major Depression Interface

The patients we now call "borderlines" were commonly referred to as *ambulatory* or *pseudoneurotic schizophrenics* in the 1930s, 1940s, and 1950s (Deutsch 1942; Grinker et al. 1968; Stern 1938; Zilboorg 1941). These terms alluded to the fact that the "psychotic" features in these patients tended to be transient or fleeting in nature. As studies characterizing the phenomenology of borderline patients emerged in the 1960s and 1970s, a prominent affective component was consistently reported, leading many clinicians to view BPD as having a close relationship to depression (Akiskal 1981; Akiskal et al. 1985a; Gunderson and Elliott 1985; Klein 1977; Stone 1980). The affective symptoms commonly seen in borderline patients included affect instability, boredom, and suicidal ideation.

The concept that BPD represents a variant of depression has been put forth by Gunderson and Elliott (1985) and more recently by Gunderson and Phillips (1991) as one of several testable hypotheses to explain the overlap of symptoms between these two disorders. In accordance with this hypothesis, despair, feelings of worthlessness, poor self-esteem, suicide attempts, and unstable relationships in BPD are all seen as outgrowths of a chronic untreated affective disorder. Symptoms such as drug use, sexual promiscuity, and impulsive acts theoretically represent attempts to temporarily relieve the underlying primary disturbances in mood, although this acting-out behavior can also be seen as an attempt to relieve anxiety. Implicit in this formulation is the expectation that successful treatment of the primary mood disorder will lead to a normalization of pathological character traits and behaviors.

Previous Biological Studies of the Borderline–Major Depression Interface

Over the last 10–15 years, a number of different psychological approaches have been used to investigate the relationship between BPD and depression. The two disorders have been compared and contrasted with regard to comorbidity (Akiskal 1981; Barasch et al. 1985; Friedman et al. 1983; Fyer et al. 1988; Gaviria et al. 1982; Kroll et al. 1981; Perry and Cooper 1985; Pfohl et al. 1984; Pope et al. 1983; Shea et al. 1987; Tyrer et al. 1983; Zanarini et al. 1989), phenomenology (Blatt and Shichman 1983; Carpenter et al. 1977; Frank et al. 1987; Grinker et al. 1968; Gunderson 1977; Gunderson and Kolb 1978; Gunderson et al. 1975; Pilkonis 1988; Westen et al. 1992), family prevalence (Akiskal et al. 1985b; Baron et al. 1985; Coryell and Zimmerman 1989; Links et al. 1988; Loranger et al. 1982; Pope et al. 1983; Soloff and Millward 1983; Zanarini et al. 1988), course of illness (Pope et al. 1983; Werble 1970), and pathogenesis (Akiskal 1981; Bradley 1979; Stone 1980). Only relatively recently, however, have biological studies been performed in this patient group (e.g., reviewed by Korzekwa et al. 1993; Lahmeyer et al. 1989). The initial impetus for these studies was the explosion of information concerning the biological basis of mood disorders in the 1970s and 1980s. With the advent of neurobiological techniques that could probe a wide variety of important physiological and biological parameters, it became possible to address the interface of BPD and depression from a biological perspective (see the introduction to this volume).

Initial studies had as their supposition that biological alterations in BPD would be similar to those observed in major depression. Indeed, the first few studies performed in this area showed marked similarities between patients with BPD and those with major depression in several putative biological markers for endogenous depression. Investigators reported the presence of biological abnormalities with greater frequency in BPD than in nonpsychiatric populations. These findings included moderate to high rates of nonsuppression on the dexamethasone suppression test (DST) (Baxter et al. 1984; Beeber et al. 1984; Carroll et al. 1981; Krishnan et al. 1984; Silk et al. 1985; Soloff et al. 1982; Sternbach et al. 1983), altered thyroid-stimulating hormone responses to thyroid-releasing hormone (Garbutt et al. 1983; Nathan et al. 1986; Sternbach et al. 1983), and shortened latencies of rapid eye movement sleep (Akiskal et al. 1985b; Bell et al. 1983; King et al. 1987; Lahmeyer et al. 1988; McNamara et al. 1984; Reynolds et al. 1985; Silk et al. 1988).

Whereas there was general agreement in these studies that biological alterations were present in patients with BPD, it was difficult to evaluate the extent to which the biological alterations observed truly reflected the biological basis of BPD, or rather, the co-occurrence of major depression (Gold and Silk 1993). Indeed, in cases where significant differences were present between BPD patients and other groups, many investigators attributed the alterations observed to the comorbidity of major depression in the borderline patients under study (Beeber et al. 1984; Bell et al. 1983; Carroll et al. 1981; Garbutt et al. 1983; King et al. 1987; Lahmeyer et al. 1988, 1989; McNamara et al. 1984; Reynolds et al. 1985; Sternbach et al. 1983). In cases where BPD could be differentiated from major depression, such as in studies reporting low rates of nonsuppression on the DST (Nathan et al. 1986; Silk et al. 1988), borderline patients could not be differentiated from healthy control subjects.

In our studies, we have observed differences in measures of catecholamine metabolism between patients with BPD and those with MDD. Moreover, we have found significant differences between BPD patients and nonpsychiatrically ill control subjects. As will be described below, this approach has been successful largely because the biological measures utilized are not primarily related to mood disorders per se, but rather, have a wider range of variation across psychiatric and other disorders. This range of variation permits a wider discrimination and an increased ability to assess the extent to which the biology of BPD differs from that of MDD and the extent to which it might be similar to that of other conditions.

Biological Discrimination Between Borderline Personality Disorder and Major Depression Through Selection of a Relevant Marker

In the first experiment, we selected platelet MAO activity to study the extent to which patients with BPD would show biological alterations similar to those of depressed patients. Platelet MAO activity is currently considered a genetically determined trait marker that may indicate a general constitutional vulnerability, or risk factor, for the development of psychopathology. However, it should be noted that activity of platelet MAO has been found to be altered (i.e., increased or decreased) in response to a variety of situations (Buchsbaum et al. 1976; Haier et al. 1980; Pandey et al. 1980; Siever and Coursey 1985; Yehuda et al. 1987). The study of platelet MAO activity in BPD was chosen not as an attempt to explore the pathophysiology of BPD, but rather, as an attempt to differentiate BPD from major depression.

Platelet MAO activity has been found to be increased in MDD (Gudeman et al. 1982; Wahlund et al. 1983). We reasoned that if biological abnormalities in borderline pathology reflected a co-occurring major depression, as suggested by several investigators, then platelet MAO activity should be increased in BPD as well. Increased platelet MAO activity in BPD would follow the trend of the research discussed above, wherein biological abnormalities in BPD resembled those seen in major depression. On the other hand, low MAO activity had been associated with personality characteristics such as sensation seeking (Demisch et al. 1982; Donnelly et al. 1979; Fowler et al. 1980; Murphy et al. 1977; Schooler et al. 1978; von Knorring et al. 1984), impulsivity (Perris et al. 1980; Schalling et al. 1987), suicidality (Buchsbaum et al. 1977; Gottfries et al. 1980), psychopathy (Lidberg et al. 1985), substance abuse (Major and Murphy 1978; Stillman et al. 1978), and perceptual aberrations (Yehuda et al. 1987) in nonpsychotic subjects. Given the similarities between many of these characteristics and the symptoms of BPD, it was also possible that platelet MAO activity would be decreased in this disorder. Furthermore, a preliminary study by Lahmeyer et al. (1988) found decreased MAO levels in borderline patients with high lithium ratios. Thus, measurements of platelet MAO activity allowed us to test the hypothesis that the biology of BPD may in fact be separate and distinct from that of major depression.

Indeed, platelet MAO activity was found to be significantly lower in a sample of 15 nonpsychotic male patients with BPD when compared with nonpsychiatrically ill control subjects (Figure 4–1; Yehuda et al. 1989). Of further importance is that there was no relationship between MAO activity level and depression scores on the Hamilton Rating Scale for Depression (HRSD; Hamilton 1960), nor were there significant differences in MAO activity when the borderline group was subdivided into those meeting and not meeting criteria for concurrent major depression. Thus, by using a biological measure that has shown a wide range of variability in different psychiatric illnesses, we were able

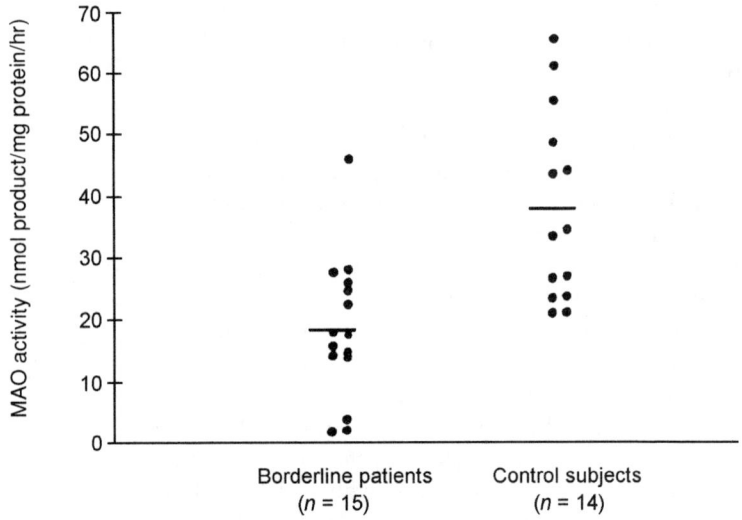

Figure 4–1. Platelet MAO activity in male patients with BPD and nonpsychiatric control subjects.
Note. Mean ± SD = 18.9 ± 11.6, 38.34 ± 15.3, for BPD patients and control subjects, respectively ($t = 3.86$, df = 27, $P < .001$).
Source. Reprinted from Yehuda R, Southwick SM, Edell WS, et al: "Low Platelet Monoamine Oxidase Activity in Borderline Personality Disorder." *Psychiatry Res* 30:268, 1989. Used with permission.

to differentiate BPD from MDD. Our results differed from those reported by Lahmeyer et al. (1988), who attributed low MAO activity in borderline patients to a comorbid Axis I disorder; however, they were subsequently replicated by Reist et al. (1990).

Because MAO activity is essential in the turnover of biogenic amines, these findings led us to further examine peripheral catecholamine metabolism in BPD.

STUDIES OF PLATELET ALPHA$_2$-ADRENERGIC ACTIVITY IN BORDERLINE PERSONALITY DISORDER

The findings of low platelet MAO activity in BPD led us to initiate a series of studies comparing platelet alpha$_2$-adrenergic receptor binding in BPD and MDD (Southwick et al. 1990b). Alpha$_2$-adrenergic receptors are relevant to an understanding of catecholamine metabolism because they are one of the receptors that mediate postsynaptic adrenergic activity and also inhibit norepinephrine release from presynaptic terminals (Perry and U'Prichard 1984). Alpha$_2$-adrenergic receptors in platelets and nervous tissue share pharmacological properties (e.g., agonist/antagonist binding affinities, inhibitory coupling to adenylate cyclase) (Bylund and U'Prichard 1983). Thus, many investigators have studied platelet alpha$_2$-adrenergic receptors as a way to evaluate changes in catecholamine metabolism.

Although there were no prior reports of platelet alpha$_2$-adrenergic receptor binding in borderline patients, several laboratories had already studied platelet alpha$_2$-adrenergic receptor binding in MDD. The results of these studies were not consistent. Some laboratories reported an increase in platelet alpha$_2$-adrenergic receptor binding (Doyle et al. 1985; Garcia-Sevilla et al. 1981, 1986, 1987; Healy et al. 1983; Kafka and Paul 1986; Pandey et al. 1989; Piletz and Halaris 1988; Siever et al. 1984), others reported a decrease in receptor number (Carstens et al. 1986; Wood et al. 1985), and still others reported no difference in receptor number (Campbell et al. 1985; Cooper et al. 1985; Daiguji et al. 1981; Georgotas et al. 1987; Lenox et al. 1983; Pimoule et al. 1983; Stahl et al. 1983; Wolfe et al. 1987). The discrepancies among studies were most often attributed to differences in biochemical methodology such as tissue preparation, choice of radioligand, or range of concentrations for saturation studies (Garcia-Sevilla et al. 1986; Kafka and Paul 1986; Kafka et al. 1986; Perry and U'Prichard 1984).

In our investigation of platelet alpha$_2$-adrenergic receptor binding, we utilized the selective alpha$_2$ antagonist ^{3}H-rauwolscine (Perry and U'Prichard 1984). Full Scatchard analyses with an extended range of concentrations (0.12 nM–35 nM) of rauwolscine were used to detect the presence of both low- and high-affinity states of the alpha$_2$-adrenergic receptor. The assay utilized was developed by Perry and U'Prichard and is described in detail elsewhere (Perry and U'Prichard 1984; Southwick et al. 1990a, 1990b). Briefly, frozen platelet pellets were thawed, sonicated, then washed with ice-cold Tris containing 50 nM ethylenediaminetetraacetic acid (EDTA), pH 7.7, and then again with Tris and 50 nM sodium chloride, pH 7.7. The final pellet was resuspended in 50 nM Tris buffer (pH 7.7 at 40°C). Total binding of ^{3}H-rauwolscine was measured in 0.3-ml aliquots of platelet membrane suspension that were incubated with 12 concentrations of the ligand for 45 minutes at 25°C. Specific binding was defined as that inhibited by 100 µM (-)-norepinephrine (in 0.1% ascorbic acid). Incubation was terminated by rapid filtration over Whatman GF/B filters. The radioactivity remaining in the filters was measured with liquid scintillation spectrometry. Receptor binding was expressed as number of binding sites per platelet. The interassay coefficient of variation for repeat determinations from the same sample was 12%. To determine the number of receptors per platelet, untransformed raw data were analyzed using a data reduction program (EBDA; McPherson 1985) that ultimately determines whether the data are best fit by a single-site or a two-site model. (For a more comprehensive discussion of the importance of assessing the two alpha$_2$-adrenergic binding sites in psychiatric disorders, see Southwick et al. [1990a, 1990b] and Perry et al. [1990].)

A Scatchard analysis provides information about the affinity of the receptor for the ligand, expressed as K_d (or dissociation constant), as well as an estimate of the total number of receptor binding sites (B_{max}). This type of analysis also affords the opportunity of detecting multiple binding sites if they are present. Scatchard analyses are typically performed to analyze experiments in which a constant number of receptors (i.e., in a standardized volume of tissue) is incubated with incremental concentrations of radioactive ligand. As the concentration of the ligand increases, more receptors can become "bound" to the ligand. As more receptors become bound to the ligand, fewer "free" receptors remain available. Eventually, the concentration of the ligand will be sufficiently high to "saturate" the receptors, and at this point adding more ligand will not result in increased binding of the drug to the receptor. The concentration at which saturation occurs defines the "affinity" of the ligand (K_d) for the receptor; K_d differs based on the pharmacological properties of the particular ligand. Once this dose-response information is obtained, the data can be subjected to further analysis. In a Scatchard analysis, the number of bound receptors is plotted against the number of bound/free receptors. The two "intercepts" generated by the plot estimate the number of binding sites per molecule (B_{max}) and the slope of the line that is equivalent to 1/(equilibrium dissociation constant [K_d]), respectively.

Study 1: Investigation of Alpha$_2$-Adrenergic Receptor Binding in Depressed Patients With and Without BPD

We first examined platelet alpha$_2$-adrenergic receptor binding in patients meeting criteria for MDD who met or did not meet criteria for BPD. All patients were evaluated for Axis I disorders with the Schedule for Affective Disorders and Schizophrenia (SADS; Endicott and Spitzer 1978). Patients were also interviewed with the Diagnostic Interview for Borderlines (DIB; Gunderson et al. 1981) to determine whether they met DIB criteria for BPD. Of the 23 patients who met Research Diagnostic Criteria (RDC; Spitzer et al. 1978) for MDD, 15 also met criteria for BPD.

When all patients with MDD ($n = 23$) were considered as one group, there were no significant differences between patients ($n = 23$) and control subjects ($n = 25$) in the affinity (K_d) for either rauwolscine binding site or in the total number of rauwolscine binding sites (B_{max}). Patients with depression did show a signifi-

Table 4–1. Platelet alpha$_2$-adrenergic receptor binding sites in major depressive disorder (MDD) patients with and without BPD and in nonpsychiatric control subjects (Study 1)

	Site 1				Site 2				Total receptor sites/platelet		Ratio site 1/site 2	
	K_d(nM)		B_{max}		K_d(nM)		B_{max}					
	Mean	SD	Mean	SD	Mean	SD	Mean	SD	Mean	SD	Mean	SD
Controls ($n = 25$)	0.40	0.17	26.1	10.0	28.3	9.1	189.9	58.5	216.1	61.0	14.4	5.9
Total MDD group ($n = 23$)	0.40	0.20	39.4[a]	24.5	24.7	8.1	186.9	111.8	226.3	129	22.9[d]	12.4
MDD + BPD ($n = 15$)	0.40	0.20	28.6	16.7	22.5	6.2	118.6[b]	37.2	147.1[c]	45.5	24.4[d]	13.6
MDD ($n = 8$)	0.30	0.27	59.9[a]	24.5	28.81	10.0	315.1[b]	88.0	375.0[c]	97.6	20.1[d]	9.9

[a]$F = 5.56$, df $= 2,39$, $P < .007$ (site 1). Total MDD versus controls was also significant. Post hoc testing revealed that only MDD alone was significantly different from controls.
[b]$F = 6.18$, df $= 2,39$, $P < .005$ (site 2). Total MDD versus controls was not significant. Significant difference was between MDD alone and controls.
[c]$F = 6.78$, df $= 2,39$, $P < .003$ (total sites [site 1 + site 2]). Total MDD versus controls was not significant. Significant difference was between MDD alone and controls.
[d]$F = 3.44$, df $= 2,39$, $P < .04$ (ratio of affinity sites [site 1/site 2]). Significance remained regardless of whether the MDD group was subdivided.

cant increase in the number of rauwolscine high-affinity sites (site 1 receptors), and consequently a significantly higher ratio of high- to low-affinity binding sites (site 1/site 2) (Table 4–1).

When the depressed patients were subdivided into two groups based on the presence or absence of comorbid BPD, patients with major depression alone ($n = 8$) had 60% more total rauwolscine binding sites compared with nonpsychiatrically ill control subjects, whereas patients with depression and BPD ($n = 15$) had 30% fewer total binding sites compared with control subjects (Figure 4–2). The results also suggested that patients with BPD were biologically different from patients with MDD, even though the BPD patients also met diagnostic criteria for major depression.

The finding of an increased number of alpha$_2$-adrenergic binding sites in the depressed patients was consistent with several previous reports (Doyle et al. 1985; Garcia-Sevilla et al. 1981, 1986, 1987; Healy et al. 1983; Kafka and Paul 1986; Pandey et al.

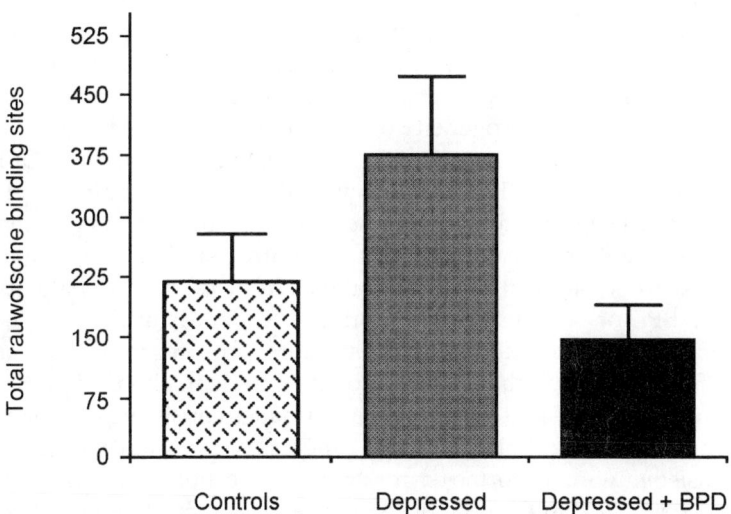

Figure 4–2. Platelet alpha$_2$-adrenergic receptor binding sites in depressed patients with and without BPD and in nonpsychiatric control subjects (Study 1).

1989; Piletz and Halaris 1988; Siever et al. 1984). This finding in the periphery (platelets) potentially reflects altered central nervous system (CNS) alpha$_2$-adrenergic receptor dysfunction. Therefore, it is possible that an increased number of alpha$_2$ binding sites results in an increased inhibition of norepinephrine release from the locus coeruleus neurons and a subsequent decrease in the amount of norepinephrine in the synaptic cleft (Charney et al. 1981; Garver and Zemlan 1986). The finding of increased alpha$_2$-adrenergic receptor binding was also consistent with studies of platelet alpha$_2$-adrenergic receptor responsiveness that showed a decreased ability of norepinephrine to inhibit prostaglandin E–stimulated cyclic adenosine monophosphate (cAMP) in depressed patients with a dysregulated receptor system (Siever et al. 1984).

Our findings were also consistent with studies that found no differences in alpha$_2$-adrenergic receptor binding sites between patients with major depression and other groups (Campbell et al. 1985; Cooper et al. 1985; Daiguji et al. 1981; Georgotas et al. 1987; Lenox et al. 1983; Pimoule et al. 1983; Stahl et al. 1983; Wolfe et al. 1987). Although, as stated above, methodological differences in assay characteristics have been thought to account for discrepancies between laboratories in the ability to observe consistent changes in the alpha$_2$-adrenergic receptor, our results raised the possibility that heterogeneity of subject populations may also be an important contributor to the inconsistencies observed. Our findings suggested that studies in which differences in alpha$_2$-adrenergic receptor binding were not observed between depressed patients and nonpsychiatrically ill control subjects may have failed to separate depressed patients from depressed patients with BPD or perhaps other comorbid disorders as well.

The finding of a decreased alpha$_2$-adrenergic receptor number in BPD suggested that unlike depressed patients, borderline patients may have a catecholamine disturbance consisting of a long-term "hypercatecholaminemia," whereas depression would be consistent with a shorter-term change in catecholamines. Indeed, a lower density of alpha$_2$-adrenergic receptor binding sites had been reported in several chronic stress disorders, such as congestive heart failure (Weiss et al. 1983), PTSD (Perry et al. 1987, 1990), and panic anxiety (Cameron et al. 1984), each of which is characterized by increased catecholamine activity. Long-lasting catecholamine alterations are consistent with the idea that BPD is a stable and enduring condition marked by chronic distress.

Study 2: Investigation of Platelet Alpha$_2$-Adrenergic Receptor Binding in Nondepressed BPD Patients

In Study 1, all patients met the diagnostic criteria for MDD. Thus, even though patients with comorbid BPD had a smaller number of alpha$_2$-adrenergic receptors, it was not clear whether nondepressed borderline patients would show differences in platelet alpha$_2$-adrenergic receptor number when compared with nonpsychiatric control subjects.

In a second study, we explored this question by studying 24 patients with BPD who did not meet RDC for major depression and 18 nonpsychiatric control subjects. Thirteen of the patients were medication free at the time of biological testing. Eleven were being treated acutely with moderate doses of benzodiazepines at the time of blood drawing: four patients were receiving chlordiazepoxide (25, 50, 40, and 75 mg/day, respectively), three were receiving temazepam (15, 15, and 45 mg/day), one was receiving 15 mg/day of diazepam, one was receiving 0.5 mg/day of alprazolam, one was receiving both 75 mg/day of chlordiazepoxide and 1.5 mg/day of alprazolam, and one was receiving both 50 mg/day of chlordiazepoxide and 30 mg/day of temazepam. Severity of depressive symptoms at the time of the drawing of blood was determined with the HRSD. The age- and sex-comparable control group ($n = 18$) was medication free and had no history of psychiatric illness or substance abuse as assessed by the SADS.

The results of this study are presented in Table 4–2. As indicated, there were no group differences in the affinity (K_d) of ^{3}H-rauwolscine for either site 1 or site 2 receptors. Nonmedicated patients with BPD had a significantly lower number of total (site 1 + site 2) rauwolscine binding sites compared with both control subjects and BPD patients being treated with benzodiazepines. There were no significant differences in the total number of binding sites in the medicated borderline patients and the control subjects; however, the medicated borderline patients had a significantly higher number of site 1 rauwolscine binding sites compared with both nonmedicated borderline patients and control subjects (Yehuda et al. 1988).

From a clinical point of view, it was of interest that the nonmedicated borderline patients were indistinguishable from benzodiazepine-treated borderline patients in their mean HRSD scores, even though they showed a significantly different number of adrenergic receptors. The mean ± standard deviation (SD) HRSD score of the nonmedicated borderline patients was 23.3 ± 10.6, and that of the medicated borderline patients was 27.5 ± 12.1 ($t = 0.88$, df = 21, not significant). When items 8 and 9 (corresponding to psychic and somatic anxiety symptoms) of the HRSD were summed and averaged, the nonmedicated borderline patients reported a 58% higher anxiety score than did the medicated borderline patients (2.69 ± 0.52 versus 1.7 ± 0.52, respectively) ($t = 1.32$, df = 21, not significant). Regression analysis of all patients with BPD failed to reveal any significant correlation between the number of binding sites and the anxiety measures from the HRSD. However, when the borderline subgroups were considered separately, there was a significant correlation between the number of alpha$_2$-adrenergic binding sites and the anxiety scores on the HRSD in the nonmedicated borderline patients ($r = .56$, df = 12, $P < .05$).

These findings extended the results of Study 1 in demonstrating that lower numbers of alpha$_2$-adrenergic receptors are present in nondepressed, as well as depressed, borderline patients. Examination of the mean number of binding sites in borderline patients from both studies revealed that the presence of MDD did not affect the number of alpha$_2$-adrenergic binding sites in patients with BPD, nor was there a relationship between the number of alpha$_2$-adrenergic binding sites and scores on the HRSD. Indeed, what appeared more closely allied to the number of alpha$_2$-adrenergic receptors in borderline patients was symptoms of anxiety as measured on the HRSD. This fact was supported by the statistically significant difference in site 1 and site 2 receptors between benzodiazepine-treated and nontreated patients with BPD, and also by the significant positive correlation between anxiety symptoms and alpha$_2$-adrenergic binding sites in the nonmedicated group.

Table 4–2. Platelet alpha$_2$-adrenergic binding measures in medicated and nonmedicated patients with BPD and in nonpsychiatric control subjects (Study 2)

	Site 1				Site 2				Total receptor sites/platelet[c]	
	K_d(nM)		B_{max}[a]		K_d(nM)		B_{max}[b]			
	Mean	SD	Mean	SD	Mean	SD	Mean	SD	Mean	SD
Nonmedicated patients with BPD ($n = 13$)	0.34	0.17	22.0	11.7	22.4	4.0	120.3[d]	50.1	142.3[d]	56.0
Medicated patients with BPD ($n = 11$)	0.40	0.22	41.9[e]	22.0	26.7	8.9	198.6	88.0	240.5	89.9
Control subjects ($n = 18$)	0.39	0.17	26.9	9.6	25.5	8.6	192.4	63.7	219.3	67.4

[a]There was a significant difference among the three groups ($F = 6.18$, df $= 2,39$, $P < .005$).
[b]There was a significant difference among the three groups ($F = 5.56$, df $= 2,39$, $P < .007$).
[c]There was a significant difference among the three groups ($F = 6.78$, df $= 2,39$, $P < .003$).
[d]Significantly lower than both the control subjects and the medicated BPD patients ($P < .05$, Newman-Keuls post hoc test).
[e]Significantly greater than both the nonmedicated BPD patients and the control subjects ($P < .05$, Newman-Keuls post hoc test).

The findings from this second platelet alpha$_2$ study led us to examine more closely the relationship between alpha$_2$-adrenergic binding sites and anxiety in benzodiazepine- and non-benzodiazepine-treated borderline patients.

Study 3: Investigation of Platelet Alpha$_2$-Adrenergic Receptor Number in Unmedicated and Benzodiazepine-Treated BPD Patients

The results of Study 2 suggested that it would be of interest to perform repeat determinations of platelet alpha$_2$-adrenergic receptor binding sites with the same subjects. Repeat examination would accomplish the objective of assessing the stability of platelet alpha$_2$-receptor binding sites in nonmedicated individuals and also of determining whether the same borderline patients would show a different number of alpha$_2$-adrenergic receptors depending on whether or not they were currently being treated with benzodiazepines. Because the research was being conducted over a 3-year period at the Brief Treatment Evaluation Unit of the Psychiatry Service at the West Haven Veterans Administration Medical Center (West Haven, Connecticut), and because many patients treated on this unit were referred to the hospital's mental hygiene clinic for continued treatment, it was possible to obtain longitudinal data for some of these individuals.

We examined 15 borderline patients and 7 nonpsychiatrically ill control subjects at two separate times. There were no significant differences in either K_d or B_{max} for any of the binding sites between the times of the first and second assessments in both cohorts—the 7 control subjects and the 8 nonmedicated borderline patients. The borderline patients did show a substantially higher number of platelet alpha$_2$-adrenergic receptors when they were being treated with benzodiazepines than when they were medication free (Figure 4–3).

This study provided support for the observation that benzodiazepine-treated borderline patients are less anxious than non-medicated patients, and that borderline patients have a greater number of platelet alpha$_2$-adrenergic receptors when they are medicated with benzodiazepines than when they are medication

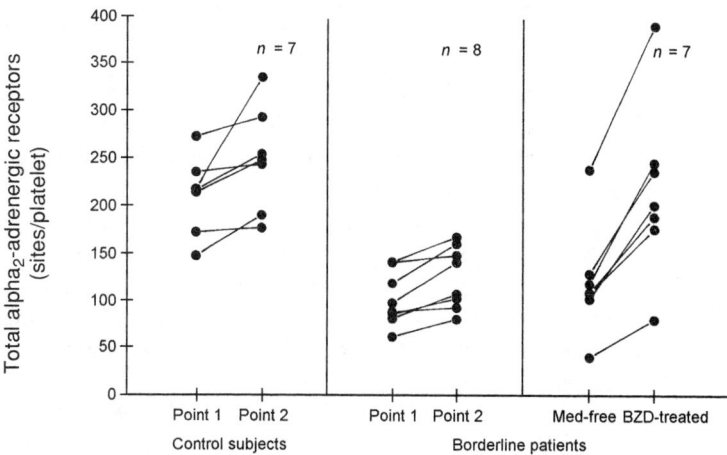

Figure 4–3. Platelet alpha$_2$-adrenergic receptor number in unmedicated and benzodiazepine-treated patients with BPD and in nonpsychiatric control subjects (Study 3).
Note. In the control and the unmedicated borderline groups, point 1 represents the estimate of the lowest number of binding sites, and point 2 the highest number of binding sites for the patient specified. In the third panel, borderline patients are presented while medication free and benzodiazepine (BZD) treated.

free. The platelet alpha$_2$-adrenergic receptor number in benzodiazepine-treated borderline patients was comparable to the number found in nonpsychiatrically ill control subjects.

It should be mentioned that the direct effects of benzodiazepines at alpha$_2$-adrenergic receptors are fairly minimal (Perry and U'Prichard 1984), and it is likely that the effects at the alpha$_2$-adrenergic receptor are indirect. Nonetheless, these "indirect" effects appear to be related to anxiety, since there were no differences between medicated and nonmedicated patients in severity of depression or in overall symptoms.

That alpha$_2$-adrenergic receptors appear to reflect anxiety symptoms in BPD can be understood in the context of the substantial literature on catecholamines and anxiety. Although a detailed examination of this relationship is beyond the scope of this review, it is noteworthy that substantial evidence exists for both peripheral and central noradrenergic overactivity in anxiety (see, for example, Redmond and Huang 1979; Uhde et al. 1984). Furthermore, drugs that specifically bind to alpha$_2$-adrenergic receptors have well-established effects on fear behaviors in animals and on anxiety in humans (Redmond 1987). Clonidine, an alpha$_2$-adrenergic agonist, has anxiolytic properties, whereas yohimbine, a specific alpha$_2$-adrenergic antagonist, has anxiogenic properties. One possible explanation for these findings is that the benzodiazepines interact with central noradrenergic systems and decrease sympathetic activity. Thus, in these "anxious" patients, benzodiazepine treatment may have decreased overall peripheral sympathetic activity.

CONCLUSIONS

Taken together, the studies of catecholamine metabolism in BPD that have been reviewed in this chapter do not support the hypothesis that BPD is a subtype or variant of depression. Instead, catecholamine metabolism in patients with BPD appears to resemble catecholamine metabolism seen in anxious patients. Lending further support to this notion is the finding of similar changes in the number of alpha$_2$-adrenergic receptors in combat veterans with chronic PTSD (Perry et al. 1987). PTSD is classified as an anxiety disorder in DSM-III-R (American Psychiatric Association 1987). Furthermore, like BPD, PTSD has been shown to be phenomenologically distinct from major depression. BPD has recently been conceptualized as a traumatic stress response disorder related to chronic childhood physical or sexual abuse, a concept that has construct validity (Herman 1992) and that has been supported by retrospective studies that reveal high frequencies of childhood abuse in patients with BPD compared with patients with other psychiatric disorders (Herman et al. 1989; Ogata et al. 1990; van der Kolk et al. 1991). A comparison of patients with BPD and individuals with PTSD appears warranted. The fact that catecholamine metabolism in BPD is similar to that in PTSD in preliminary studies may reflect the role that chronic stress and trauma appear to play in the etiology of many symptoms found in these disorders.

REFERENCES

Akiskal HS: Subaffective disorders: dysthymic, cyclothymic and bipolar II disorders in the "borderline" realm. Psychiatr Clin North Am 4:25–46, 1981

Akiskal HS, Chen SE, David GC, et al: Borderline: an adjective in search of a noun. J Clin Psychiatry 46:41–48, 1985a

Akiskal HS, Yerevanian BI, Davis GC, et al: The nosologic status of borderline personality: clinical and polysomnographic study. Am J Psychiatry 142:192–198, 1985b

American Psychiatric Association: Diagnostic and Statistical Manual of Mental Disorders, 3rd Edition, Revised. Washington, DC, American Psychiatric Association, 1987

Barasch A, Frances A, Hurt S, et al: Stability and distinctness of borderline personality disorder. Am J Psychiatry 142:1484–1486, 1985

Baron M, Gruen R, Asnis L et al: Familial transmission of schizotypal and borderline personality disorders. Am J Psychiatry 142:927–934, 1985

Baxter L, Edell W, Gerner R, et al: Dexamethasone suppression test and Axis I diagnoses of inpatients with DSM-III borderline personality disorder. J Clin Psychiatry 45:150–153, 1984

Beeber AR, Kline MD, Pies RW, et al: Dexamethasone suppression test in hospitalized depressed patients with borderline personality disorder. J Nerv Ment Dis 172:301–303, 1984

Bell J, Lycaki H, Jones D, et al: Effect of preexisting borderline personality disorder on clinical and EEG sleep correlates of depression. Psychiatry Res 9:115–123, 1983

Blatt SJ, Shichman S: Two primary configurations of psychopathology. Psychoanalysis and Contemporary Thought 6:187–254, 1983

Bradley SJ: The relationship of early maternal separation to borderline personality in children and adolescents: a pilot study. Am J Psychiatry 136:424–426, 1979

Buchsbaum MS, Coursey RD, Murphy DL: The biochemical high risk paradigm: behavioral and familial correlates of low platelet MAO activity. Science 194:339–341, 1976

Buchsbaum MS, Haier RJ, Murphy DL: Suicide attempts, platelet monoamine oxidase and the average evoked response. Acta Psychiatr Scand 56:69–79, 1977

Bylund DB, U'Prichard DC: Characterization of $alpha_1$- and $alpha_2$-adrenergic receptors. Int Rev Neurobiol 24:343–431, 1983

Cameron OG, Smith CB, Hollingsworth PJ, et al: Platelet alpha$_2$-adrenergic receptor binding and plasma catecholamine: before and during imipramine treatment in patients with panic anxiety. Arch Gen Psychiatry 41:1144–1148, 1984

Campbell IC, McKernana RM, Checkley SA, et al: Characterization of platelet alpha$_2$-adrenoreceptors and measurement in controls and depressed subjects. Psychiatry Res 14:17–31, 1985

Carpenter WT, Gunderson JG, Strauss JS: Considerations of the borderline syndrome: a longitudinal comparative study of borderline and schizophrenic patients, in Borderline Personality Disorders. Edited by Hartocollis P. New York, International Universities Press, 1977, pp 231–253

Carroll BJ, Greden JF, Feinberg M, et al: Neuroendocrine evaluation of depression in borderline patients. Psychiatr Clin North Am 4:89–99, 1981

Carstens ME. Engelbrecht AH, Russell VA, et al: Alpha$_2$-adrenoreceptor levels on platelets of patients with major depressive disorders. Psychiatry Res 18:321–331, 1986

Charney DS, Heninger GR, Sternberg DE, et al: Presynaptic adrenergic receptor sensitivity in depression: the effect of long-term desipramine treatment. Arch Gen Psychiatry 38:1334–1339, 1981

Cooper SJ, Kelly JG, King DJ: Adrenergic receptors in depression: effects of electroconvulsive therapy. Br J Psychiatry 147:23–29, 1985

Coryell WH, Zimmerman M: Personality disorder in the families of depressed, schizophrenic, and never ill probands. Am J Psychiatry 146:496–502, 1989

Daiguji M, Meltzer HY, Tong C, et al: Alpha$_2$-adrenergic receptor in platelet membranes of depressed patients: no change in number of ^{3}H yohimbine affinity. Life Sci 29:2059–2064, 1981

Demisch L, Georgi K, Patzke B, et al: Correlation of platelet MAO activity with introversion: a study on a German rural population. Psychiatry Res 6:303–311, 1982

Deutsch H: Some forms of emotional disturbance and their relationship to schizophrenia. Psychoanal Q 11:301–321, 1942

Donnelly EF, Murphy DL, Waldman IN, et al: Psychological characteristics corresponding to low versus high platelet monoamine oxidase activity. Biol Psychiatry 14:375–383, 1979

Doyle MC, George AJ, Ravindran AV: Platelet alpha$_2$-adrenoreceptor binding in elderly depressed patients. Am J Psychiatry 142:1489–1490, 1985

Endicott J, Spitzer RL: A diagnostic interview: the schedule for affective disorders and schizophrenia. Arch Gen Psychiatry 35:837–844, 1978

Fowler CJ, von Knorring L, Oreland L: Platelet monoamine oxidase activity in sensation seekers. Psychiatry Res 3:273–279, 1980

Frank E, Kupfer DJ, Jacob M, et al: Personality features and response to acute treatment in recurrent depression. Journal of Personality Disorders 1:13–26, 1987

Friedman RC, Aronoff MS, Clarkin JF, et al: History of suicidal behavior in depressed borderline patients. Am J Psychiatry 140:1023–1026, 1983

Fyer MR, Frances AJ, Sullivan T, et al: Comorbidity of borderline personality disorder. Arch Gen Psychiatry 45:349–352, 1988

Garbutt JC, Loosen PT, Tipermas A, et al: The TRH test in patients with borderline personality disorder. Psychiatry Res 9:107–113, 1983

Garcia-Sevilla JA, Zis AP, Hollingsworth PJ, et al: Platelet alpha$_2$-adrenergic receptors in major depressive disorder. Arch Gen Psychiatry 38:1327–1333, 1981

Garcia-Sevilla JA, Guimon J, Garcia-Vallejo P, et al: Biochemical and functional evidence of supersensitive platelet alpha$_2$-adrenoreceptors in major affective disorder: effect of long-term lithium carbonate treatment. Arch Gen Psychiatry 43:51–57, 1986

Garcia-Sevilla JA, Udina C, Fuster MJ, et al: Enhanced binding of ^{3}H-(-)adrenaline to platelets of depressed patients with melancholia: effect of long-term clomipramine treatment. Acta Psychiatr Scand 75:150–157, 1987

Garver DL, Zemlan FP: Receptor studies in diagnosis and treatment of depression, in Depression: Basic Mechanisms, Diagnosis and Treatment. Edited by Rush AJ, Altshuler KZ. New York, Guilford, 1986, pp 143–170

Gaviria M, Flaherty J, Val E: A comparison of bipolar patients with and without a borderline personality disorder. Psychiatr J Univ Ottawa 7:190–195, 1982

Georgotas A, Schweitzer J, McCue RE, et al: Clinical and treatment effects on ^{3}H-clonidine and ^{3}H-imipramine bindings in elderly depressed patients. Life Sci 40:2137–2143, 1987

Gold LJ, Silk KR: Exploring the borderline personality disorder–major affective disorder interface, in Borderline Personality Disorder: Etiology and Treatment. Edited by Paris J. Washington, DC, American Psychiatric Press, 1993, pp 39–66

Gottfries C, von Knorring L, Oreland L: Platelet monoamine oxidase activity in mental disorders, II: affective psychoses and suicidal behavior. Progress in Neuro-Psychopharmacology 4:185–192, 1980

Grinker RR, Werble B, Drye RC: The Borderline Syndrome: A Behavioral Study of Ego Functions. New York, Basic Books, 1968

Gudeman JE, Schatzberg AF, Samson JA, et al: Toward a biochemical classification of depressive disorders, VI: platelet MAO activity and clinical symptoms in depressed patients. Am J Psychiatry 139:630–633, 1982

Gunderson JG: Characteristics of borderlines, in Borderline Personality Disorder: The Concept, The Syndrome, The Patient. Edited by Hartocollis P. New York, International Universities Press, 1977, pp 173–192

Gunderson JG, Elliott GR: The interface between borderline personality disorder and affective disorder. Am J Psychiatry 142:277–288, 1985

Gunderson JG, Kolb JE: Discriminating features of borderline patients. Am J Psychiatry 135:792–796, 1978

Gunderson JG, Phillips KA: A current view of the interface between borderline personality disorder and depression. Am J Psychiatry 148:967–975, 1991

Gunderson JG, Sabo AN: The phenomenological and conceptual interface between borderline personality disorder and PTSD. Am J Psychiatry 150:19–27, 1993

Gunderson JG, Carpenter WT, Strauss JS: Borderline and schizophrenic patients: a comparative study. Am J Psychiatry 132:1257–1264, 1975

Gunderson JG, Kolb JE, Austin V: The Diagnostic Interview for Borderline Patients. Am J Psychiatry 138:896–903, 1981

Haier RJ, Buchsbaum MS, Murphy DL, et al: Psychiatric vulnerability, monoamine oxidase, and the average evoked potential. Arch Gen Psychiatry 37:340–345, 1980

Hamilton M: A rating scale for depression. J Neurol Neurosurg Psychiatry 23:56–62, 1960

Healy D, Carney PA, Leonard BE: Monoamine related markers of depression: changes following treatment. J Psychiatric Res 17:251–260, 1983

Herman JL: Complex PTSD: a syndrome of survivors of prolonged and repeated trauma. Journal of Traumatic Stress 5:377–391, 1992

Herman JL, Perry JC, van der Kolk BA: Childhood trauma in borderline personality disorder. Am J Psychiatry 146:490–495, 1989

Kafka MS, Paul SM: Platelet alpha$_2$-adrenergic receptors in depression. Arch Gen Psychiatry 43:91–95, 1986

Kafka MS, Nurnberger JI, Siever L, et al: Alpha$_2$-adrenergic receptor function in patients with unipolar and bipolar affective disorders. J Affective Disord 10:163–169, 1986

King R, Benson KL, Zarcone VP: REM latency in borderlines and depressed. Sleep Research 16:280, 1987

Klein DF: Psychopharmacological treatment and delineation of borderline disorders, in Borderline Personality Disorders: The Concept, The Syndrome, The Patient. Edited by Hartocollis P. New York, International Universities Press, 1977, pp 365–384

Korzekwa M, Links P, Steiner M: Biological markers in borderline personality disorder: new perspectives. Can J Psychiatry 36 (suppl 1, Feb):1–5, 1993

Krishnan KR, Davidson JRT, Rayasam K, et al: The dexamethasone suppression test in borderline personality disorder. Biol Psychiatry 19:1149–1153, 1984

Kroll J, Sines L, Martin K, et al: Borderline personality disorder: construct validity of the concept. Arch Gen Psychiatry 38:1021–1026, 1981

Lahmeyer HW, Val E, Gaviria M, et al: EEG sleep, lithium transport, dexamethasone suppression and monoamine oxidase activity in borderline personality disorder. Psychiatry Res 25:19–30, 1988

Lahmeyer HW, Reynolds CF III, Kupfer DJ, et al: Biologic markers in borderline personality disorder: a review. J Clin Psychiatry 50:217–225, 1989

Lenox RH, Ellis J, Van Riper DA, et al: Platelet alpha$_2$-adrenergic receptor activity in clinical studies of depression, in Frontiers in Neuropsychiatric Research. Edited by Usdin E, Goldstein M, Friedhoff A. New York, Macmillan, 1983, pp 331–356

Lidberg L, Modin I, Oreland L, et al: Platelet monoamine oxidase activity and psychopathy. Psychiatry Res 16:339–343, 1985

Links PS, Steiner M, Huxley G: The occurrence of borderline personality disorder in the families of borderline patients. Journal of Personality Disorders 2:14–20, 1988

Loranger AW, Odham JM, Tulis EH: Familial transmission of DSM-III borderline personality disorder. Arch Gen Psychiatry 39:795–799, 1982

Major LF, Murphy DL: Platelet and plasma amine oxidase activity in alcoholic individuals. Br J Psychiatry 132:548–554, 1978

McNamara E, Reynolds CF III, Soloff PH, et al: EEG sleep evaluation of depression in borderline patients. Am J Psychiatry 141:182–186, 1984

McPherson GA: Kinetic, EBDA, LIGAND, Lowry: A Collection of Radioligand Binding Analysis Programs, Manual. Amsterdam, Elsevier Biosoft, 1985

Murphy DL, Belmaker RH, Buchsbaum MS, et al: Biogenic amine-related enzymes and personality variation in normals. Psychol Med 7:149–157, 1977

Nathan RS, Soloff PH, George A, et al: DST and TRH tests in borderline personality disorder, in Biological Psychiatry: Proceedings of the 4th World Congress of Biological Psychiatry. Edited by Shagass C, Josiassen RG, Wagner BH, et al. New York, Elsevier, 1986, pp 564–565

Ogata SN, Silk KR, Goodrich S, et al: Childhood sexual and physical abuse in adult patients with borderline personality disorder. Am J Psychiatry 147:1008–1013, 1990

Pandey GN, Dorus E, Shaughnessy R, et al: Reduced platelet MAO activity and vulnerability to psychiatric disorders. Psychiatry Res 2:315–321, 1980

Pandey GN, Janicak PG, Javiad JI, et al: Increased ^{3}H-clonidine binding in the platelets of patients with depressive and schizophrenic disorders. Psychiatry Res 28:73–88, 1989

Perris C, Jacobsson L, von Knorring L, et al: Enzymes related to biogenic amine metabolism and personality characteristics in depressed patients. Acta Psychiatr Scand 61:477–484, 1980

Perry JC, Cooper SH: Psychodynamics, symptoms, and outcome in borderline and antisocial personality disorders and bipolar type II affective disorder, in The Borderline: Current Empirical Research. Edited by McGlashan TH. Washington, DC, American Psychiatric Press, 1985, pp 19–41

Perry BD, U'Prichard DC: ^{3}H-rauwolscine (alpha-yohimbe): a specific antagonist radioligand for brain alpha$_2$-adrenergic receptors. Eur J Pharmacol 76:462–464, 1981

Perry BD, U'Prichard DC: Alpha-adrenergic receptors in neural tissues: methods and application of radiological binding assays, in Brain Receptor Methodologies, Part A: General Methods and Concepts. Edited by Marangos PJ, Campbell IC, Cohen RM. New York, Academic Press, 1984, pp 256–284

Perry BD, Giller EL, Southwick SM: Altered platelet alpha$_2$-adrenergic binding sites in post-traumatic stress disorder. Am J Psychiatry 144:1511–1512, 1987

Perry BD, Southwick SM, Yehuda R, et al: Adrenergic receptor regulation in posttraumatic stress disorder, in Biological Assessment and Treatment of Posttraumatic Stress Disorder. Edited by Giller EL. Washington, DC, American Psychiatric Press, 1990, pp 89–114

Pfohl B, Stangl D, Zimmerman ML: The implications of DSM-III disorders for patients with major depression. J Affective Disord 7:309–318, 1984

Piletz JE, Halaris AG: Super high affinity ^{3}H-para-aminoclonidine binding to platelet adrenoreceptors in depression. Prog Neuropsychopharmacol Biol Psychiatry 12:541–553, 1988

Pilkonis PA: Personality prototypes among depressives: themes of dependency and autonomy. Journal of Personality Disorders 2:144–154, 1988

Pimoule C, Briley MS, Gay C, et al: ^{3}H-rauwolscine binding in platelet from depressed patients and healthy volunteers. Psychopharmacology (Berl) 79:308–312, 1983

Pope HG, Jonas JM, Hudson JI, et al: The validity of DSM-III borderline personality disorder: A phenomenologic, family history, treatment response, and long-term follow-up study. Arch Gen Psychiatry 40:23–30, 1983

Redmond DE Jr: Studies of the nucleus locus coeruleus in monkeys and hypotheses for neuropsychopharmacology, in Psychopharmacology: The Third Generation of Progress. Edited by Meltzer HY. New York, Raven, 1987, pp 967–975

Redmond DE Jr, Huang YH: Current concepts, II: new evidence for a locus coeruleus–norepinephrine connection with anxiety. Life Sci 25:2149–2162, 1979

Reist C, Haier RJ, DeMet E, et al: Platelet MAO activity in personality disorders and normal controls. Psychiatry Res 33:221–227, 1990

Reynolds CF III, Soloff PH, Kupfer DJ, et al: Depression in borderline patients: a prospective EEG sleep study. Psychiatry Res 14:1–15, 1985

Schalling D, Åsberg M, Edman G, et al: Markers for vulnerability to psychopathology: temperament traits associated with platelet MAO activity. Acta Psychiatr Scand 76:172–182, 1987

Schooler C, Zahn TP, Murphy DL, et al: Psychological correlates of monamine oxidase activity in normals. J Nerv Ment Dis 166:177–186, 1978

Shea MT, Glass DR, Pilkonis PA: Frequency and implications of personality disorders in a sample of depressed outpatients. Journal of Personality Disorders 1:27–42, 1987

Siever LJ, Coursey RD: Biological markers for schizophrenia and the biological high-risk approach. J Nerv Ment Dis 173:4–16, 1985

Siever LJ, Kafka MS, Targum S, et al: Platelet alpha-adrenergic binding and biochemical responsiveness in depressed patients and controls. Psychiatry Res 11:287–302, 1984

Silk KR, Lohr NE, Cornell DG, et al: The dexamethasone suppression test in borderline and nonborderline affective patients, in The Borderline: Current Empirical Research. Edited by McGlashan T. Washington, DC, American Psychiatric Press, 1985, pp 99–116

Silk KR, Lohr NE, Shipley JE, et al: Sleep EEG and DST in borderlines with depression. Paper presented at the 141st annual meeting of the American Psychiatric Association, Montreal, Canada, May 1988

Soloff PH, Millward JW: Psychiatric disorders in the families of borderline patients. Arch Gen Psychiatry 40:37–44, 1983

Soloff PH, George A, Nathan R: Dexamethasone suppression test in patients with borderline personality disorder. Am J Psychiatry 139:1621–1622, 1982

Southwick SM, Yehuda R, Giller EL, et al: Altered platelet alpha$_2$-adrenergic binding sites in borderline personality disorders. Am J Psychiatry 147:1014–1017, 1990a

Southwick SM, Yehuda R, Giller EL, et al: Platelet alpha$_2$-adrenergic receptor binding sites in major depressive disorder and borderline personality disorder. Psychiatry Res 34:193–203, 1990b

Spitzer RL, Endicott J, Robins E: Research diagnostic criteria: rationale and reliability. Arch Gen Psychiatry 35:773–782, 1978

Stahl SM, Lemoine PM, Ciaranello RD, et al: Platelet alpha$_2$-adrenergic receptor sensitivity in major depressive disorder. Psychiatry Res 10:157–164, 1983

Stern A: Psychoanalytic investigation of and therapy in the borderline group of neuroses. Psychoanal Q 7:467–489, 1938

Sternbach HA, Fleming J, Extein I, et al: The dexamethasone suppression and thyrotropin-releasing hormone test in depressed borderline patients. Psychoneuroendocrinology 8:459–462, 1983

Stillman RC, Wyatt R, Murphy DL, et al: Low platelet monoamine oxidase activity and chronic marijuana use. Life Sci 23:1577–1581, 1978

Stone MH: The Borderline Syndromes: Constitution, Adaptation and Personality. New York, McGraw-Hill, 1980

Tyrer P, Casey P, Gall J: Relationship between neurosis and personality disorder. Br J Psychiatry 142:404–408, 1983

Uhde TW, Boulenger JP, Post RM, et al: Fear and anxiety: relationship to noradrenergic function. Psychopathology 3 (suppl 17):8–23, 1984

van der Kolk BA, Perry JC, Herman JL: Childhood origins of self-destructive behavior. Am J Psychiatry 148:1665–1671, 1991

von Knorring L, Oreland L, Winblad B: Personality traits related to monoamine oxidase activity in platelets. Psychiatry Res 12:11–16, 1984

Wahlund LO, Smedy Y, Saag J, et al: Influence of hemodialysis on monamine oxidase kinetics in platelets from chronic schizophrenic patients. Artif Organs 7:334–339, 1983

Weiss RT, Tobes M, Wertz CE, et al: Platelet alpha$_2$-adrenoceptors in chronic congestive heart failure. Am J Cardiol 52:101–105, 1983

Werble B: Second follow-up study of borderline patients. Arch Gen Psychiatry 23:3–7, 1970

Westen D, Moses J, Silk KR, et al: Quality of depressive experience in borderline personality disorder and major depression: when depression is not just depression. Journal of Personality Disorders 6:382–393, 1992

Wolfe N, Coehn BM, Gelenberg AJ: Alpha$_2$-adrenergic receptors in platelet membranes of depressed patients: increased affinity for ^{3}H-yohimbine. Psychiatry Res 20:107–116, 1987

Wood K, Swade C, Coppen A: Platelet alpha-adrenergic receptors in depression: ligand binding and aggregation studies. Acta Pharmacologica et Toxicologica 1 (suppl 56):203–11, 1985

Yehuda R, Edell WS, Meyer JS: Platelet MAO activity and psychosis proneness in college students. Psychiatry Res 20:129–132, 1987

Yehuda R, Perry BD, Southwick SM, et al: Alpha$_2$-adrenergic binding following benzodiazepine treatment in borderline personality disorder. Society for Neuroscience Abstracts 14:412, 1988

Yehuda R, Southwick SM, Edell WS, et al: Low platelet monoamine oxidase activity in borderline personality disorder. Psychiatry Res 30:265–273, 1989

Zanarini MC, Gunderson JG, Marino MF, et al: DSM-III disorders in the families of borderline outpatients. Journal of Personality Disorders 2(4):292–302, 1988

Zanarini MC, Gunderson JG, Frankenburg FR: Axis I phenomenology of borderline personality disorder. Compr Psychiatry 30:149–156, 1989

Zilboorg G: Ambulatory schizophrenia. Psychiatry 4:149–155, 1941

Chapter 5

Borderline Personality Disorder and the Anxiety Disorders

Kenneth R. Silk, M.D.
JoAnn Goodson, B.S.N., M.P.H.
Jane Benjamin, Ph.D.
Naomi E. Lohr, Ph.D.

Current research in borderline personality disorder (BPD) has paid much less attention to exploring the relationship of BPD to the anxiety disorders than it has to investigating the relationship between BPD and the affective disorders (Gunderson and Elliott 1985; Gunderson and Phillips 1991). This is true despite the fact that for more than 40 years psychodynamic formulations have emphasized the function of borderline symptoms as a possible mechanism for binding anxiety (Grotstein 1984).

In 1959, while defining the concept of "pseudoneurotic schizophrenia," a probable early synonym for patients with mixed borderline and schizotypal features, Hoch and Cattell noted that

> there is a low threshold to the anxiety response, with a low threshold to experiencing it, and bewilderment in coping with it. An anxiety response may occur in reaction to neutral or minimally threatening stimuli. Situations or stimuli that are ordinarily reassuring may provoke anxiety. Anxiety may occur in association with any change in the immediate situation in which the patient finds himself, or with any change in his activity or location. The anticipation of anything new is especially threatening and new experiences are usually avoided unless someone else takes the initial steps and serves as convoy. (p. 32)

They further pointed out that

> actually there is diffuse anxiety in almost every area of behavior. This anxiety seems impervious to every effort for relief made by the patient or his environment. Patients are often bewildered in trying to account for this inexplicable anxiety. (Hoch and Cattell 1959, p. 33)

Almost 15 years later, in describing patients with borderline personality organization, Kernberg (1975) wrote the following:

> Such patients tend to present chronic, diffuse, free-floating anxiety. This symptom becomes particularly meaningful when a variety of other symptoms or pathological character traits are present. The anxiety, therefore, exceeds the binding capacity of the other symptoms and character traits.... Multiple phobias, especially those which impose severe restrictions on the patient's daily life... [and] those involving severe social inhibitions and paranoid trends, are presumptive evidence of borderline personality organization. (p. 9)

In the earliest papers in which the term *borderline* was used, the idea of lack of regulation and tolerance of anxiety was viewed as a significant aspect of the clinical picture. Stern (1938) believed that anxiety arose whenever borderline patients were faced with a demand to function as adults. Moreover, Stern thought that the anxiety, although connected to a strong sense of insecurity, seemed to be related to constitutional as well as psychological factors. Grinker et al. (1968), in their empirical study of the borderline concept, divided the borderline diagnosis into four subgroups. Whereas anxiety, particularly the anxiety related to separation, was important in each of the subgroups, Group IV patients, often depicted as anxious and phobic, were described as seeming to be pushed back and forth by anxiety; if these patients moved too close to an object, their anxiety and anger would drive them back (or drive the object away); if they moved too far away from an object, the anxiety of separation would motivate them back toward the object.

Other analytically oriented authors, from Masterson (1976) to Adler and Buie (1979) to Meissner (1984), have referred to anxiety in the borderline group of patients, particularly as it manifests itself in the treatment setting. In this setting, anxiety frequently appears related to fears of annihilation—annihilation resulting from loss of identity and/or merging (or the wish to merge) with the therapist. Not unlike the situation described by Grinker et al., this anxiety appeared to buffet the borderline patient between the wish for merger with its accompanying terror of engulfment and annihilation on the one hand and the pain and suffering of loneliness and isolation, of frustration of one's narcissistic needs, on the other.

Despite references throughout the analytic and dynamic literature to the role of anxiety in the borderline syndromes, there is scant mention of anxiety among our current diagnostic criteria for BPD. While Gunderson and Singer (1975) considered anxiety as a possible defining affect, they rejected its inclusion in their criteria set because they felt that it was "difficult in most instances to know if [the anxiety being described was] a symptomatic problem among borderline patients or [if the other authors of the papers they were reviewing were] making an inference based on a theoretical role given anxiety in personality theories" (p. 4). In Gunderson and Singer's first criterion—the presence of intense affect—they list anger and depression, leaving only the idea of depersonalization as perhaps being connected or related to anxiety symptoms.

This discounting of anxiety symptoms continued in the official DSM-III and DSM-III-R diagnoses of borderline personality disorder (American Psychiatric Association 1980, 1987). In DSM-III, anxiety is referred to as a manifestation of affective instability only in the phrase "marked shifts from normal mood to depression, irritability, or anxiety, usually lasting a few hours and only rarely more than a few days, with a return to normal mood" (American Psychiatric Association 1980, p. 323).

The role of anxiety in or the relationship of the anxiety disorders to BPD remains an area in need of further exploration. The debate of the early 1980s with respect to the relationship between BPD and affective disorders seems to have quieted (Gunderson and Phillips 1991; Gold and Silk 1993). Recent research into the biology of aggression and suicide has brought much attention to the role of impulsivity in BPD. This relationship is elaborated more fully in Chapters 1 and 2 of this volume (see also Zanarini 1993). Sexual and physical abuse and other early childhood traumatic experiences have attracted intense interest with respect to their role in the etiology or the particular symptomatic profile of the borderline patient (Herman and van der Kolk 1987; Ogata et al. 1990; Westen et al. 1990; Zanarini et al. 1989b). In fact, the recent interest in trauma and BPD, and in issues related to the differential diagnosis between BPD and posttraumatic stress disorder (PTSD) (Gunderson and Sabo 1993), can be viewed as a reawakening of interest in anxiety and its relationship to BPD since 1) PTSD is classified in DSM under the anxiety disorders, and 2) dissociative episodes, which have often been part of the borderline picture in the past and are included in the borderline criteria set in DSM-IV (American Psychiatric Association 1994; Gunderson et al. 1991), seem closely related not only to trauma but also to panic or other severe anxiety states.

A surprisingly high percentage of patients with Axis I disorders also have a concurrent Axis II disorder, and the diagnostic co-occurrence of Axis I anxiety disorders and Axis II personality disorder, with particular attention to BPD and the other dramatic cluster personality disorders (histrionic, narcissistic, and antisocial), will be reviewed here. Koenigsberg et al. (1985) found that 46% of 1,932 patients (both inpatients and outpatients) with an Axis I diagnosis also had a concurrent personality disorder diagnosis. In this study, 50% of panic patients and 48% of phobic patients met criteria for a personality disorder—particularly borderline, histrionic, dependent, or mixed for the panic patients, and avoidant, dependent, mixed, or histrionic for the phobic subjects. More specifically, 12% (4/32) of the panic disorder patients also met the borderline diagnosis; 25% (8/32) of the panic patients—or 20% of all subjects with anxiety disorders (panic, phobic, general, and atypical anxiety disorder)—also met criteria for a dramatic cluster diagnosis.

Studies that specifically looked at Axis II diagnoses in Axis I anxiety disorder patients found that almost 45% of anxiety patients had a concurrent Axis II disorder. Those anxiety disorder subjects with a concurrent personality disorder did more poorly, had a worse prognosis, and had a higher frequency of dependent personality disorder. Reich et al. (1987), using the Structured

Interview for DSM-III Personality Disorders (SIDP; Stangl et al. 1985), found that 6/88 (7%) of their panic patients met BPD criteria and 13/88 (15%) met criteria for one of the dramatic cluster personality disorders. They found poor outcome with respect to panic symptomatology among those patients who also met dramatic cluster personality disorder criteria. Interestingly, the panic in these poor-outcome subjects was primarily reactive or situational rather than the spontaneous panic usually found in classical panic disorder. Friedman et al. (1987) found that 58% of 26 panic disorder patients also met criteria for at least one DSM-III personality disorder (as assessed with a preliminary version of the Structured Clinical Interview for DSM-III-R Axis II Personality Disorders [SCID-II; Spitzer et al. 1990]). While only one met borderline criteria, 25% met criteria for at least one of the dramatic cluster diagnoses. Nurnberg et al. (1989), using the LEAD (Longitudinal Expert Evaluation using all Data) method (Skodol et al. 1988), found that 15% (9/62) of anxiety disorder patients also met BPD criteria, and Mavissakalian et al. (1990), using the Personality Diagnostic Questionnaire (PDQ; Hyler et al. 1988), found that 3 (2%) of 187 panic patients met the criteria for BPD, with 29 (16%) meeting the criteria for some dramatic cluster diagnosis. Using the SCID-II, Green and Curtis (1988), on the other hand, found no borderline patients and only 2 (8%) dramatic cluster patients among a cohort of 25 panic disorder patients. It is interesting to note that the two studies that used the SCID-II for personality disorder diagnoses, Friedman et al. (1987) and Green and Curtis (1988), found very low frequencies of BPD among panic patients, whereas studies using other instruments for Axis II diagnoses often found a much higher frequency.

Curiously, most borderline patients who meet criteria for panic disorder and/or generalized anxiety disorder (GAD) also meet criteria for an affective disorder. Grunhaus et al. (1985) found that 36% of 28 borderline inpatients met Research Diagnostic Criteria (RDC; Spitzer et al. 1978) for panic disorder, and all of the 36% also met criteria for major depressive disorder. Zanarini et al. (1989a) found that among 50 outpatients who met DSM-III and Diagnostic Interview for Borderlines (DIB; Gunderson at al. 1981) criteria for BPD, 78% met SCID criteria for major depression and 100% met criteria for dysthymia. Further, 24%

met criteria for GAD, 16% for panic disorder (one subject here also had agoraphobia), and 10% for simple phobia. Weiler et al. (1988) found that among 21 borderline inpatients, 57% met criteria for panic disorder, and 66% of the panic disorder subgroup also met criteria for major depression. In this latter study, the borderline patients who also met criteria for panic disorder had more current symptoms, more diagnoses, more symptoms in childhood (especially separation anxiety), and more separation experiences during childhood. Akiskal (1981) found that 13 of 100 DSM-III borderline outpatients met criteria for either panic or agoraphobia, while Bell et al. (1983) found that borderline patients who were depressed had more symptoms of panic, phobia, and general anxiety than did depressed subjects without BPD.

This co-occurrence of anxiety and depressive symptoms in borderline patients may perhaps relate to the fact that borderline patients' depression is often primarily atypical (Parsons et al. 1989), an admixture of anxiety and depression. Or this finding may be, in some senses, artifactual, since the Schedule for Affective Disorders and Schizophrenia (SADS; Endicott and Spitzer 1978) and the RDC—the Axis I structured interview schedules in most frequent use during the 1980s in the United States—were biased toward the diagnosis of affective disorder over anxiety disorder. Rather than allowing patients to be comorbid for both anxiety and affective disorder, the SADS and the RDC strongly directed the diagnosis toward affective disorder categories. Perhaps many borderline patients, particularly if they entered the hospital with suicidal ideation or suicide attempts, were first seen as having both depression and BPD. As the treating psychiatrist became more familiar with a patient, he or she became more aware of anxiety symptoms and then added an anxiety diagnosis to the affective diagnosis. If this reasoning is correct, it is conceivable that there are many borderline patients who were, because of this diagnostic idiosyncrasy, classified as comorbid for affective disorder when in fact the comorbidity may have been with the anxiety disorders. In our follow-up study of 24 borderline subjects, 3 of the 4 subjects with anxiety disorder diagnoses on follow-up had had affective disorder diagnoses (without anxiety disorder diagnoses) on index 2–4 years previously (Silk et al. 1991).

Pharmacological response in borderline patients may provide further clues to the role of anxiety in BPD. Some borderline patients appear to have a better response to the monoamine oxidase inhibitors (MAOIs) than to the tricyclics (Cowdry and Gardner 1988; Soloff et al. 1993). MAOIs are known to be effective not only in panic disorder but in atypical and anxious depression as well (Parsons et al. 1989), and the effectiveness of MAOIs in borderline patients may be related to this mixture of anxious and depressive symptomatology (Liebowitz et al. 1984).

There are other clinical phenomena that occur among borderline patients that may indirectly relate to anxiety. Studies that have explored transient psychotic episodes in borderline patients often attribute the psychosis to a temporary regression triggered by anxiety. Chopra and Beatson (1986) found dissociative phenomena (derealization and/or depersonalization) in 92% of their 13 subjects. Seven had "brief" psychotic experiences (paranoid, depressive, or drug-induced) that were often relieved through supportive measures. These transient psychoses were attributed to "intense anxiety resulting from the patients' inability to cope with their stresses, particularly in unstructured situations" (Chopra and Beatson 1986, p. 1606). Gunderson (1984) believes that borderline patients' fluctuating clinical pictures may result from anxiety related to actual or fantasized object loss. As anxiety about potential or actual object loss increases, the patient switches his or her psychological level of functioning, resulting in different clinical pictures and defensive functioning at each of three different levels. This anxiety resulting from either anticipation of or actual separation may contribute to the confusing and ever-changing "stable instability" (Schmideberg 1947) in the clinical picture of these patients.

Our population of borderline inpatients at the University of Michigan almost universally present with depressive symptoms. The reasons they enter the hospital are most often related to suicidal ideation or suicide attempts, gestures, or threats that often occur in response to interpersonal crises. In about half of the patients, the depression fails to meet DSM-III criteria for a major depressive episode and frequently falls into the diagnostic category of dysthymia or adjustment disorder with depressed mood.

Yet even though these hospitalized patients talk about suicide and make suicidal attempts or gestures, these actions do not always—and perhaps even do not usually—occur because of depressed affect. Frequently, patients who cut or otherwise mutilate themselves do so not because of depression but because of severe feelings of detachment or depersonalization and the extreme anxiety that accompanies these states. The cutting often represents an attempt to create pain so as to organize themselves and define their own boundaries (Leibenluft et al. 1987). Self-mutilators often feel relieved and much less anxious after cutting, but soon the anxiety and tension that lead to dissociation begin to build again, thus perpetuating the cycle of tension elevation, dissociation, cutting, and tension reduction, and eventually leading again to new tension elevation.

Borderline patients who enter the hospital may complain of depressive symptomatology, but they also report anxiety symptoms. Although these patients often use the word "panic" to describe their anxiety, the "panic attack" they describe is atypical. It seems more situational, related to or triggered by social situations. The attack appears to last anywhere from a few moments to perhaps an hour and often is accompanied by feelings of depersonalization and/or derealization. It is in the context of this "panic" or during prolonged periods of dissociation that borderline patients not only self-mutilate but also abuse substances and engage in promiscuous behavior. These maneuvers appear to be attempts to quell the panic. Even though these panics may be atypical, they can lead to suicide and other disturbing behaviors (Allgulander and Lavori 1991; Johnson et al. 1990).

Of the 89 borderline subjects in our cohort (Silk et al. 1989), 52% readily admit to episodes of depersonalization or derealization, with an additional 22% reporting milder or less identifiable dissociative experiences. Seventy-three percent admit to severe symptoms of psychic or somatic anxiety (from the Hamilton Rating Scale for Depression [Hamilton 1960]) or severe symptoms of dissociation (from the DIB). Forty-five percent report severe psychological anxiety, while 27% report severe somatic anxiety (from the Hopkins Symptom Checklist—90 [SCL-90; Derogatis et al. 1974]). Twenty percent acknowledge both severe psychic and somatic anxiety, and 10% admit to not only severe psychic and somatic anxiety but definite and frequent dissociative episodes as well. These percentages are not dissimilar to those of other studies reported above, wherein somewhere between 10% and 25% of borderline patients meet criteria for and/or report significant symptoms related to panic and/or anxiety.

Few studies have explored biological correlates or measures of anxiety in borderline patients. Yehuda, Southwick, and Reiser have done most of the work in this area, and their studies are summarized in Chapter 4. To review one study for the purposes of this chapter, Southwick et al. (1990) found a significant decrease in platelet alpha$_2$-adrenergic binding sites among unmedicated borderline patients compared with either medicated borderline patients or nonpsychiatrically ill control subjects, with the unmedicated borderline patients having an average somatic and psychic anxiety score 58% higher than those of the other two groups. The authors suggest that this decrease in binding sites may be related to chronic overexposure to catecholamines, a theory that has been used to explain the decrease in alpha$_2$-adrenergic binding sites among PTSD patients as well as panic disorder patients. Southwick and colleagues suggest that, compared with medicated BPD patients and control subjects, unmedicated borderline patients experience greater anxiety and probably greater chronic sympathetic arousal.

In order to more fully explore anxiety in BPD, we chose to utilize a test for a putative biological marker for a predisposition to panic attacks. Sodium lactate has been used for the last 20 years as a pharmacological probe for panic (Pitts and McClure 1967). It is beyond the scope of this chapter to review in detail the literature on lactate infusion; the reader is referred to the article by Cowley and Arana (1990), who conclude that panic induced by sodium lactate infusion has a 67% sensitivity and an 87% specificity in differentiating patients with panic from nonpsychiatric control subjects. Lactate infusion can provoke panic in 56% of psychiatric patients with panic attacks but in only 10% of patients without panic attacks. Cowley and Arana also conclude that whereas lactate-induced panic is not specific for the diagnosis of panic disorder, it is specific for the presence of panic attacks irrespective of the comorbid diagnosis.

LACTATE INFUSION IN BORDERLINE PATIENTS

Methods

All subjects were drawn from two inpatient units at the University of Michigan Medical Center. Potential borderline subjects met at least two criteria for DSM-III BPD or schizotypal personality disorder (SPD) on admission. Subjects were screened to exclude patients with ongoing medical problems that would preclude participation in a drug-free period or that would confound biological test results.

There were many more subjects willing to participate in the noninvasive parts of our protocol than were willing to undergo the lactate infusion. While approximately 82% of eligible subjects agreed to participate in our broader study, only 25% of that 82% agreed to the lactate infusion. Those who consented to any part of the study were then administered the DIB during the drug-free period by a research team member. Interrater reliability for the DIB (0.78) by our group has been published elsewhere (Cornell et al. 1983), and reliability has been maintained through periodic retraining and assessment. RDC and DSM-III-R diagnoses were made by consensus of the patient's primary therapist and a senior supervisor. No one who administered the DIB to a given patient was involved in that patient's RDC diagnosis.

The sodium lactate infusion was carried out under a single-blind condition, and the protocol used for the infusion follows the procedure of Sheehan et al. (1985). The procedure was carried out in the patient's own room. After an angiocath was inserted in the patient's arm, a solution of 5% dextrose in normal saline was infused over 30 minutes at the rate of 100cc/hour. The infusate was then changed to a 0.5 molar racemic solution of sodium lactate in normal saline. A total volume of 10cc/kg of body weight of that 0.5M solution was then infused over the next 20–25 minutes. During the entire procedure, a research nurse and a physician were present. The patient was told that the rater physician did not know whether the second solution was an active solution or placebo. The research nurse was aware of the contents of the solution. Although the physician was, in truth, unaware of whether the solution contained sodium lactate, he or she *was* aware that the instruction given to the pharmacy was to prepare active solution much more frequently than placebo. The patient was told to talk about any feelings or sensations as they occurred, and these were recorded by the physician. Pulse and blood pressure were recorded every 15 minutes during the entire procedure. At the conclusion of the infusion, a panic symptom checklist that contained all 13 DSM-III-R symptoms of panic was filled out by the physician based on his or her discussion of each symptom with the patient and after considering all the statements made by the patient during the infusion. Each symptom was rated on a 4-point scale: absent, mild/doubtful, moderate, or severe. For a symptom to be recorded as having occurred, a rating of 3 or 4 had to be given. At the end of the period of lactate infusion, the infusate was changed back to the 5% dextrose in normal saline solution and this solution was continued for an additional 15 minutes.

Results

All seven subjects were women and ranged in age from 19 to 36. While all met both DIB and DSM-III-R criteria for BPD, none had a comorbid diagnosis of panic disorder or GAD upon admission or discharge. Additional comorbid discharge diagnoses included dysthymia ($n = 3$), antisocial personality disorder ($n = 2$), cyclothymia ($n = 1$), and SPD ($n = 1$).

Four of the seven subjects experienced a sufficient number of symptoms for us to say that they had experienced a panic attack. Three subjects experienced 7 symptoms, and one subject, 10 symptoms. Two subjects who did not experience an attack reported only 2 symptoms, and one subject only 3 symptoms.

Among the subjects who experienced an attack, the most frequently reported symptom in response to the lactate was trembling and shaking. Next most frequent was a depersonalization/derealization experience. Chest tightness and fear of going crazy were also prominent symptoms. Palpitations, dizziness, nausea and abdominal discomfort, numbness, tingling, and chills were frequently reported. Sweating or the experience of choking was never reported.

All of the subjects who met our criteria for panic claimed that they had experienced panic in the past, and all but one stated that they were still experiencing symptoms of panic close to the time of their admission. Interestingly, however, it was not the symptoms of panic or anxiety, at least outwardly, that led them to seek admission. One of the subjects who had no response to the test denied ever having experienced panic. Two of the nonresponders also acknowledged having panic attacks in the past and currently, but they denied experiencing any significant anxiety during the infusion. Three of the four responders reported the symptom of fear of going crazy or of losing control. However, they stated that the presence of the research nurse and the physician as well as the knowledge that the "attack" was being brought on by the lactate helped them to keep focus and not lose control. Two of the responders said that the feeling created by the lactate was the feeling that they tried to overcome through acts of self-mutilation.

Six of the seven subjects had a history of sexual abuse, but there was no relationship between response to lactate and any particular type or severity of sexual abuse. While Rainey et al. (1987) have been able, with sodium lactate, to induce flashbacks in Vietnam veterans with PTSD, we found no such induction of flashbacks or other images of trauma in our subjects during the infusion. All of the subjects except one returned to baseline within 15–30 minutes after the infusion. The exception was a patient who was comorbid for SPD and who vomited, had a severe headache, and felt distant and dissociated for 4–6 hours after termination of the infusion. There was no significant difference in increase in heart rate between responders and nonresponders.

Discussion

This study is clearly exploratory in nature and is ongoing. Little can be said or concluded from a study that 1) is single blind and 2) has an N of only 7. Also, because only 25% of subjects who consented to other parts of our study consented to this part, we did not have a representative sample upon which to draw conclusions. There is some sort of self-selection process here. Given that two of the responders said that the lactate induced a feeling state similar to the one they experience when they have the urge to self-mutilate, perhaps those patients who refused to participate knew very well what was at stake for them. On the other hand, one cannot state that panic patients are, in fact, any less uncomfortable at the moment of panic than are borderline patients, but perhaps, like other factors in borderline patients, the affect is, for some reason, totally intolerable and leads to some form of acting-out/self-destructive behavior.

These results do not imply that borderline patients are really misdiagnosed panic patients. As Cowley and Arana (1990) have noted, lactate-induced panic is probably not specific for the diagnosis of panic disorder but is more likely specific for the presence of panic attacks irrespective of the comorbid diagnosis. However, anxiety symptoms may be underreported by borderline patients, and these results would suggest that it is important for us to more fully explore anxiety/panic symptoms in our borderline patients. Perhaps in their everyday lives, patients with BPD do not experience anxiety symptoms in classical ways. Benjamin et al. (1989) have shown that borderline patients appear to express their anxiety with an increase in paranoia or hostility. Further, clinicians may tend to dismiss borderline patients' anxiety as "psychological," brought about by fears of separation or rejection. While this may be true, it does not rule out the possibility that these patients are also undergoing a biological event—an event that may be amenable to pharmacological treatment such as with MAOIs (Parsons et al. 1989), which have been said to be useful in the treatment of some borderline patients (Cowdry and Gardner 1988; Soloff et al. 1993).

CONCLUSIONS

We must not lose sight of the fact that for 50 years, clinicians have repeatedly described the presence and the role of anxiety in borderline states and borderline patients. Probes that have been used to explore the biology of anxiety and panic disorders in those specific diagnostic entities may find a place in the biological examination of borderline patients and those with other personality disorders. Any exploration that can shed some light on the sources and manifestations of the powerful affects that borderline patients experience and express may eventually lead to better ways to alleviate the intense affective states experienced not only among borderline patients but also among those who treat them.

REFERENCES

Adler G, Buie DH: Aloneness and borderline psychopathology: the possible relevance of child development issues. Int J Psychoanal 60:83–96, 1979

Akiskal HS: Subaffective disorders: dysthymic, cyclothymic and bipolar II disorders in the "borderline" realm. Psychiatr Clin North Am 4:25–46, 1981

Allgulander C, Lavori PW: Excess mortality among 3302 patients with "pure" anxiety neurosis. Arch Gen Psychiatry 48:599–602, 1991

American Psychiatric Association: Diagnostic and Statistical Manual of Mental Disorders, 3rd Edition. Washington, DC, American Psychiatric Association, 1980

American Psychiatric Association: Diagnostic and Statistical Manual of Mental Disorders, 3rd Edition, Revised. Washington, DC, American Psychiatric Association, 1987

American Psychiatric Association: Diagnostic and Statistical Manual of Mental Disorders, 4th Edition. Washington, DC, American Psychiatric Association, 1994

Bell J, Lycaki H, Jones D, et al: Effect of preexisting borderline personality disorder on clinical and EEG sleep correlates of depression. Psychiatry Res 9:115–123, 1983

Benjamin J, Silk KR, Lohr NE, et al: The relationship between borderline personality disorder and anxiety disorders. Am J Orthopsychiatry 59:461–467, 1989

Chopra HD, Beatson JA: Psychotic symptoms in borderline personality disorder. Am J Psychiatry 143:1605–1607, 1986

Cornell DG, Silk KR, Ludolph PS, et al: Test–retest reliability of the diagnostic interview for borderlines. Arch Gen Psychiatry 40:1307–1310, 1983

Cowdry RW, Gardner DL: Pharmacotherapy of borderline personality disorder; alprazolam, carbamazepine, trifluoperazine and tranylcypromine. Arch Gen Psychiatry 45:111–119, 1988

Cowley DS, Arana GW: The diagnostic utility of lactate sensitivity in panic disorder. Arch Gen Psychiatry 47:277–284, 1990

Derogatis LR, Lipman RS, Rickels K, et al: The Hopkins Symptom Checklist (HSCL): a self-report symptom inventory. Behav Sci 19:1–15, 1974

Endicott J, Spitzer RL: A diagnostic interview: the schedule for affective disorders and schizophrenia. Arch Gen Psychiatry 35:837–844, 1978

Friedman CJ, Shear MK, Frances A: DSM-III personality disorders in panic patients. Journal of Personality Disorders 1:132–135, 1987

Gold LJ, Silk KR: Exploring the borderline personality disorder–major affective disorder interface, in Borderline Personality Disorder: Etiology and Treatment. Edited by Paris J. Washington, DC, American Psychiatric Press, 1993, pp 39–66

Green MA, Curtis GC: Personality disorders in panic patients: response to termination of antipanic medication. Journal of Personality Disorders 2:303–314, 1988

Grinker RR, Werble B, Drye RC: The Borderline Syndrome: A Behavioral Study of Ego Functions. New York, Basic Books, 1968

Grotstein JS: A proposed revision of the psychoanalytic concept of primitive mental states, part II. Contemporary Psychoanalysis 20:77–119, 1984

Grunhaus L, King D, Greden JF, et al: Depression and panic in patients with borderline personality disorder. Biol Psychiatry 20:688–692, 1985

Gunderson JG: Borderline Personality Disorder. Washington, DC, American Psychiatric Press, 1984

Gunderson JG, Elliott GR: The interface between borderline personality disorder and affective disorder. Am J Psychiatry 142:277–288, 1985

Gunderson JG, Phillips KA: A current view of the interface between borderline personality disorder and depression. Am J Psychiatry 148:967–975, 1991

Gunderson JG, Sabo AN: The phenomenological and conceptual interface between borderline personality disorder and PTSD. Am J Psychiatry 150:19–27, 1993

Gunderson JG, Singer MT: Defining borderline patients: an overview. Am J Psychiatry 132:1–10, 1975

Gunderson JG, Kolb JE, Austin V: The Diagnostic Interview for Borderline Patients. Am J Psychiatry 138:896–903, 1981

Gunderson JG, Zanarini MC, Kisiel CL: Borderline personality disorder: a review of data on DSM-III-R descriptions. Journal of Personality Disorders 5:340–352, 1991

Hamilton M: A rating scale for depression. J Neurol Neurosurg Psychiatry 23:56–62, 1960

Herman JL, van der Kolk BA: Traumatic antecedents of borderline personality disorder, in Psychological Trauma. Edited by van der Kolk BA. Washington, DC, American Psychiatric Press, 1987, pp 111–126

Hoch PH, Cattell JP: The diagnosis of pseudoneurotic schizophrenia. Psychiatr Q 33:17–43, 1959

Hyler S, Reider R, Williams J, et al: The personality diagnostic questionnaire: development and preliminary results. Journal of Personality Disorders 2:229–237, 1988

Johnson J, Weissman MM, Klerman GL: Panic disorder, comorbidity, and suicide attempts. Arch Gen Psychiatry 47:805–808, 1990

Kernberg O: Borderline Conditions and Pathological Narcissism. New York, Jason Aronson, 1975

Koenigsberg HW, Kaplan RD, Gilmore MM, et al: The relationship between syndrome and personality disorder in DSM-III: experience with 2,462 patients. Am J Psychiatry 142:207–212, 1985

Leibenluft E, Gardner DL, Cowdry RW: The inner experience of the borderline self-mutilator. Journal of Personality Disorders 1:317–324, 1987

Liebowitz MR, Quitkin FM, Stewart JW, et al: Phenelzine versus imipramine in atypical depression: a preliminary report. Arch Gen Psychiatry 41:669–677, 1984

Masterson JF: Psychotherapy of the Borderline Adult. New York, Brunner/Mazel, 1976

Mavissakalian M, Hamann MS, Jones B: A comparison of DSM-III personality disorders in panic/agoraphobia and obsessive-compulsive disorder. Compr Psychiatry 31:238–244, 1990

Meissner WW: The Borderline Spectrum. New York, Jason Aronson, 1984

Nurnberg HG, Raskin M, Levine PE, et al: Borderline personality disorder as a negative prognostic factor in anxiety disorder. Journal of Personality Disorders 3:205–216, 1989

Ogata SN, Silk KR, Goodrich S, et al: Childhood sexual and physical abuse in adult patients with borderline personality disorder. Am J Psychiatry 147:1008–1013, 1990

Parsons B, Quitkin FM, McGrath PJ, et al: Phenelzine, imipramine, and placebo in borderline patients meeting criteria for atypical depression. Psychopharmacol Bull 25:524–534, 1989

Pitts FN, McClure JJ: Lactate metabolism in anxiety neurosis. N Eng J Med 277:1329–1336, 1967

Rainey JM, Aleem A, Ortiz A, et al: A laboratory procedure for the induction of flashbacks. Am J Psychiatry 144:1317–1319, 1987

Reich J, Noyes R Jr, Troughton E: Dependent personality disorder associated with phobic avoidance in patients with panic disorder. Am J Psychiatry 144:323–326, 1987

Schmideberg M: The treatment of psychopaths and borderline patients. Am J Psychother 1:45–55, 1947

Sheehan DV, Carr DB, Fishman SM, et al: Lactate infusion in anxiety research: its evolution and practice. J Clin Psychiatry 46:158–165, 1985

Silk KR, Cohen R, Gold L, et al: Psychotic symptoms in borderline personality disorder; consideration for DSM-IV (abstract). Biol Psychiatry 25 (suppl 7A):88A, 1989

Silk KR, Pressler EJ, Westen D, et al: Diagnostic and psychotherapeutic changes in BPD. Paper presented at the 144th annual meeting of the American Psychiatric Association, New Orleans, LA, May 1991

Skodol AE, Rosnick L, Kellman D, et al: Validating structured DSM-III-R personality disorder assessments with longitudinal data. Am J Psychiatry 145:1297–1299, 1988

Soloff PH, Cornelius J, George A, et al: Efficacy of phenelzine and haloperidol in borderline personality disorder. Arch Gen Psychiatry 50:377–385, 1993

Southwick SM, Yehuda R, Giller EL, et al: Altered platelet alpha$_2$-adrenergic binding sites in borderline personality disorders. Am J Psychiatry 147:1014–1017, 1990

Spitzer RL, Endicott J, Robins E: Research diagnostic criteria: rationale and reliability. Arch Gen Psychiatry 35:773–782, 1978

Spitzer RL, Williams JBW, Gibbon M, et al: Structured Clinical Interview for DSM-III-R Axis II Personality Disorders (SCID-II) (Version 1.0). Washington, DC, American Psychiatric Press, 1990

Stangl D, Pfohl B, Zimmerman M, et al: A structured interview for the DSM-III personality disorders: preliminary report. Arch Gen Psychiatry 42:591–596, 1985

Stern A: Psychoanalytic investigation of and therapy in the borderline group of neuroses. Psychoanal Q 7:467–489, 1938

Weiler MA, Val ER, Gaviria M, et al: Panic disorder in borderline personality disorder. Psychiatr J Univ Ottawa 13:140–143, 1988

Westen D, Ludolph P, Misle B, et al: Physical and sexual abuse in adolescent girls with borderline personality disorder. Am J Orthopsychiatry 60:55–66, 1990

Zanarini MC: BPD as an impulse spectrum disorder, in Borderline Personality Disorder: Etiology and Treatment. Edited by Paris J. Washington, DC, American Psychiatric Press, 1993, pp 67–85

Zanarini MC, Gunderson JG, Frankenburg FR: Axis I phenomenology of borderline personality disorder. Compr Psychiatry 30:149–156, 1989a

Zanarini MC, Gunderson JG, Marino MF, et al: Childhood experiences of borderline patients. Compr Psychiatry 30:18–25, 1989b

Chapter 6

Brain Imaging in Personality Disorders

Peter F. Goyer, M.D.
P. Eric Konicki, M.D.
S. Charles Schulz, M.D.

Brain imaging is a relatively new technique that is being used with increasing frequency to study neurological illnesses and psychiatric disorders. Brain imaging and other measures that attempt to "visualize" and "measure" processes and structures within the cranium have been utilized in many studies to examine groups of patients with psychiatric illnesses, but only a few of these studies have investigated a possible neuropsychiatric component to Axis II disorders. Some investigators suggest that these measures, which have been used with increasing frequency in Axis I disorders, have not been applied to personality disorders because these disorders, until recently, were thought to have primarily a psychological etiology. Others think that neuropsychiatric research was late in coming to personality disorders because of the lack of reliable and consistent diagnostic criteria.

As was noted in Chapter 5, the work of Gunderson and Singer (1975) led to the development of specific objective criteria to characterize borderline personality disorder (BPD). The advent of specific criteria allowed investigators to reliably classify BPD patients for neuropsychiatric and pharmacological studies (see the Introduction to this volume). Structured interviews were developed that could delineate BPD not only from depression and schizophrenia (Kolb and Gunderson 1980; Soloff and Ulrich 1981) but also from other personality disorders (Zanarini et al. 1989). The Diagnostic Interview for Borderlines (DIB; Gunderson et al. 1981) was able to identify the stable characteristics of patients with BPD (Frances et al. 1984). Concurrent with the development of the DIB was a refinement of the borderline diagnosis that occurred when schizotypal personality disorder (SPD) was separated out from the diagnosis of BPD (Spitzer et al. 1979). This division of the previous, broader concept of borderline personality allowed both clinicians and researchers to identify more homogeneous patient groups. The BPD patients had more symptoms of mood instability, whereas the SPD patients resembled the relatives of schizophrenic patients who had been identified and studied by Kety and his colleagues (1975) in the Danish adoption studies of the 1960s (Gunderson et al. 1983; Stone 1979).

Siever and Davis (1991) have begun to explore the boundaries of schizophrenia with an emphasis on the examination of SPD. By applying some of the research strategies used by investigators of schizophrenic disorders, they have shown that patients with schizotypy (which, for the purposes of this chapter, can be viewed as synonymous with SPD) often have research results that are quite different from those of control subjects but very similar to—and often in the same direction as—those of patients with schizophrenia. For example, plasma homovanillic acid (HVA), a dopamine metabolite, has been found to be elevated in schizotypal patients. This finding mirrors the results observed in schizophrenic patients (Siever et al. 1991). Similar abnormalities in eye tracking have been found among both schizophrenic and schizotypal patients (Siever et al. 1984). Braff (1981) found comparable information-processing impairments in both unmedicated schizotypal and schizophrenic patients. This strong relationship between SPD and schizophrenia has been further reinforced by the results of structural brain imaging studies of measures of ventricular size (Siever et al. 1987).

On the other hand, the relationship of BPD to the mood disorders remains controversial (Akiskal 1981; Gold and Silk 1993; Gunderson and Elliott 1985; Gunderson and Phillips 1991). A relationship between mood disorders and BPD appears to be supported by investigations of neuropsychiatric measures that are seen to be abnormal in depressed patients. This research has indicated that BPD patients differ from control groups in the same direction as depressed patients in dexamethasone suppression (Silk et al. 1985; Sternbach et al. 1983), sleep latency (McNamara et al. 1984), and thyroid challenge studies (Garbutt et al. 1983). However, these results are not consistent across all studies of these areas (Korzekwa et al. 1993). Reviews of the biological relationship between BPD and mood disorders are provided by Lahmeyer et al. (1989) and Korzekwa et al. (1993).

The hypothesized relationship between BPD or SPD and Axis I disorders has been explored in a number of other ways, and many of the chapters in this book provide current examples of such investigations. Some researchers have attempted to examine a battery of neuropsychiatric parameters to probe the relationship between personality disorders and Axis I disorders as well as the relationship between personality disorders and neurological disorders or dysfunction. Studies in these areas are presented and reviewed Chapters 7, 8, and 9. The work of Andrulonis et al. (1981) exemplifies this approach. Andrulonis and his colleagues reported that patients who met criteria for BPD and who also had organic brain dysfunction (e.g., minimal brain dysfunction, attention-deficit hyperactivity disorder, or learning disabilities) were "significantly distinct" from borderline patients without signs or symptoms of organic brain dysfunction. Yet here, as well, it has been difficult to consistently find groups of patients who display mild to moderate neurological abnormalities (Cornelius et al. 1989; Cowdry et al. 1985–1986; Gardner et al. 1987).

The above strategies would indicate that there is a potential role for the use of brain imaging in elucidating further the possibility of brain dysfunction in BPD and SPD. There are many studies that have used magnetic resonance imaging (MRI) and computed tomography (CT) in patients with schizophrenia. These studies reveal a number of areas in the brains of schizophrenic patients that are different from those of control subjects. It would seem appropriate, therefore, to examine ventricular size by measuring ventricular/brain ratio (VBR), absolute third ventricular size, and sulcal prominence in patients with BPD and/or SPD. Similarities and differences between the findings in these two personality disorders and the reported findings in schizophrenic patients could shed more light on the relationship among BPD, SPD, and schizophrenic disorders.

Imaging studies in populations of psychiatric patients have

not been limited only to subjects with schizophrenia. Patients with bipolar illness and depression with psychotic features have been noted to have enlarged ventricles or increased numbers of unidentified bright objects (UBOs) (Coffey et al. 1989; Dupont et al. 1987; Targum et al. 1983). Given the continuing dialogue concerning the relationship of BPD to mood disorders, it would be useful to compare the structural brain images of patients with personality disorders with those of patients with mood disorders.

One could also ignore issues of specific personality disorder diagnoses and instead concentrate on studying the brain images related to specific behaviors or dimensions that most strongly characterize patients with BPD and SPD (Cloninger 1987). The theme of dimensions of psychopathology spanning many different personality disorders has been raised repeatedly in this book. Coccaro et al. (1989), as elaborated in Chapter 2, examined the relationship between the serotonergic system and impulsivity in BPD patients, and the studies revealed significant (inverse) correlations between impulsivity and serotonin. A similar strategy could be applied to brain imaging in which behavioral dimensions, not diagnostic categories or syndromes, are used to examine pathophysiology.

In this chapter we review current work in the area of brain imaging in patients with BPD and SPD. Two recently completed studies, one in structural imaging and one in functional imaging, are described in greater depth. In the concluding section, we explore the future role of imaging studies in personality disorder research.

STRUCTURAL IMAGING—A REVIEW

Over the last decade, personality disorder patients have been targeted in imaging studies for a variety of reasons. In the earliest studies, Schulz and colleagues (Schulz et al. 1983), in their CT study of adolescents with schizophrenic disorder, used hospitalized teenage patients with BPD as a comparison group to control for the possible effects of hospitalization. In their study, the borderline patients had VBRs that were identical to those of the nonhospitalized control group and that were significantly smaller than those of the schizophrenic teenagers. Lucas and colleagues (1989), in a study comparing the effectiveness of different pharmacological agents in BPD (Cowdry and Gardner 1988), used CT to measure VBR in borderline patients; they did not find ventricular enlargement among the patients. Parnas and Teasdale (1987) examined "borderline" patients as part of a study of high-risk offspring of patients with schizophrenia. Whereas those subjects who developed schizophrenia had enlarged ventricles, the ventricles of the patients who were or who became "borderline" were smaller than not only those of the schizophrenic patients but also those of the subjects without psychiatric illness.

Siever and colleagues (1987) studied VBR in patients with SPD as part of their ongoing work to examine and clarify the relationship between SPD and schizophrenia. These investigators found that, compared with control subjects, their schizotypal patients had enlarged VBRs.

In summary, then, we find that the two studies that looked at BPD patients did not find ventricular enlargement. In fact, in one study—the high-risk study by Parnas and Teasdale (1987)—the borderline patients had smaller ventricles than even the healthy control subjects. Only the Siever et al. (1987) study, which examined schizotypal rather than borderline patients, found enlarged VBRs that were different from those of control subjects.

National Institute of Mental Health–Chestnut Lodge Study

As part of ongoing studies exploring the neuropsychiatric aspects of personality disorders, a collaborative group of investigators at the National Institute of Mental Health (NIMH) and Chestnut Lodge studied schizotypal patients who had been hospitalized for a number of years (Konicki et al. 1992). Sixteen patients (BPD = 11; SPD = 5), classified on Axis II with the Personality Disorders Examination (PDE; Loranger 1988) and on Axis I with the Schedule for Affective Disorders and Schizophrenia, Lifetime Version (SADS-L; Spitzer and Endicott 1978), were compared with six volunteers from the community. All but one of the personality disorder patients had a comorbid Axis I disorder. All subjects were rated with the Brief Psychiatric Rating Scale (BPRS; Overall and Gorham 1962).

Subjects underwent MRI scanning and an area VBR measure was developed. There was no significant difference in VBR between the patient and the control groups. However, there was a significant relationship between the VBR measure and "scores" of psychopathology in the patient group (Konicki et al. 1992). Both the total BPRS score and the total BPD score from the PDE were positively correlated with VBR. This finding suggests that within the borderline group of personality disorders, increased ventricular size may be associated with the pathophysiology of the disorder, even though the mean VBR of the patient group compared with that of the healthy control subjects was not significantly different. It is unclear how generalizable these results are, since the patients had been hospitalized for a long period of time and thus may represent a unique group of schizotypal/borderline patients.

FUNCTIONAL BRAIN IMAGING WITH POSITRON-EMISSION TOMOGRAPHY

Through the use of positron-emission tomography (PET), cerebral glucose metabolism has been studied in a number of psychotic and nonpsychotic illnesses. Illnesses studied include schizophrenia and affective disorders (Baxter et al. 1985, 1989; Buchsbaum et al. 1984; Cohen et al. 1987, 1989; Martinot et al. 1990a), panic disorder (Nordahl et al. 1990; Reiman et al. 1984, 1986), adult hyperactivity of childhood onset (Zametkin et al. 1990), obsessive-compulsive disorder (Baxter et al. 1987, 1988, 1989; Benkelfat et al. 1990; Nordahl et al. 1989; Swedo et al. 1989), summer seasonal affective disorder (Goyer et al. 1992), and posttraumatic stress disorder (Semple et al. 1993). There are also a number of studies of regional cerebral metabolic rate of glucose (rCMRG) in substance abuse. In most of the studies listed above, the rCMRG of the patient group differed significantly from that of the healthy control groups. Often, but not always, these differences occurred at various levels in the frontal cortex. Cerebral glucose metabolism and PET have begun to contribute substantially to our knowledge of psychiatric illness.

In addition to being used to study glucose metabolism, PET can be used with other radioligands, particularly radiopharmaceuticals, to obtain quantified measurements in physiological units for blood flow, oxygen metabolism, receptor density, and so forth, in specific regions of interest (ROIs). Additional data can be obtained by performing PET scans during pharmacological trials or during cognitive cerebral activation (cognitive tasks). Other functional imaging modalities, such as single photon emission computed tomography (SPECT), can be used to examine brain blood flow, but quantification in physiological units from the SPECT is more problematic than with PET, both because of controversies over models used for interpreting results and because of less-than-adequate ROI resolution. Nonetheless, SPECT coupled with cognitive activation has furthered our understanding of schizophrenia (Weinberger et al. 1986).

National Naval Medical Center–National Institute of Mental Health Study

In a collaborative PET study between the National Naval Medical Center (NNMC) and NIMH, Goyer et al. (1991) measured rCMRG in psychiatric patients diagnosed with a personality disorder. This collaboration was a continuation of an ongoing study of impulsivity, aggression, and personality disorder. Earlier studies from this two-site collaboration demonstrated that aggressivity was inversely correlated with cerebrospinal fluid (CSF) levels of the serotonin metabolite 5-hydroxyindoleacetic acid (5-HIAA) (Brown et al. 1979, 1982). This earlier work was subsequently extended to other studies that examine the role of serotonin in the impulsivity of personality disorder patients (Coccaro et al. 1990; Lidberg et al. 1985; Linnoila et al. 1983; Markovitz et al. 1991; Roy and Linnoila 1988; Virkkunen et al. 1987).

The most recent collaboration by Goyer et al. (1991) used PET and 18-fluorodeoxyglucose (^{18}FDG) to study rCMRG in a group of 17 patients with a DSM-III-R (American Psychiatric Association 1987) diagnosis of personality disorder. The patients were scanned following cortical activation with an auditory continuous performance task. This PET study found a statistically significant inverse correlation between rank on a life history of aggression scale and global CMRG ($r = -.51$, $P < .05$). Of the five transaxial planes examined, the plane approximately 40mm above the canthomeatal line (CML) showed a significant inverse correlation with group ranking and rCMRG ($r = -.62$, $P < .03$). Within this transaxial plane, absolute scores on the life history of aggression scale inversely correlated with rCMRG in three orbital frontal ROIs: right anterior frontal ($P < .05$), anterior medial frontal ($P < .03$), and left anterior frontal ($P < .05$). Of the 17 patients in the study, 6 met DSM-III-R criteria for BPD, 6 for antisocial personality disorder, and 5 for other personality disorders. Average normalized rCMRG in the 6 patients with BPD and in the 6 patients with antisocial personality disorder was compared with that of a group of 43 healthy volunteers. There were no significant differences in average normalized rCMRG between the antisocial personality disorder patients and the healthy control subjects. There were, however, significant differences in normalized rCMRG between the BPD group and the control group. In the BPD patients, there were significant decreases in average normalized rCMRG in specific ROIs in the frontal and parietal lobes of a transaxial plane approximately 81mm above the CML ($P < .05$, two-tailed t test) and a significant increase in the average normalized rCMRG in specific ROIs in the frontal lobe of a transaxial plane approximately 53mm above the CML ($P < .05$, two-tailed t test). Because of the small number of patients, replication of this study is essential to minimize the possibility of false positive findings. In addition, only 3 of the 17 patients had an unresolved Axis I diagnosis at the time of the PET study, and future studies must consider comorbid Axis I diagnoses before interpreting their results or comparing them with those of this study.

Raine et al. (1992) examined glucose metabolism in a population characterized by more severe antisocial behavior—specifically, 22 prison inmates convicted of murder. When compared with a nonpsychiatrically ill age- and sex-matched control group of 22 subjects, the convicted murderers had a statistically significant decrease in average glucose metabolic rate in the orbital frontal and prefrontal cortex. Although Goyer and colleagues (1991) did not find statistically significant differences in average rCMRG between their small number ($N = 6$) of less-severe antisocial personality disorder patients and their healthy control group, the subsequent findings of Raine et al. for mean decreases in a between-group comparison support Goyer et al.'s previously published findings of a within-group inverse correlation between a life history of difficulty with aggressive impulsivity and normalized rCMRG in the orbital frontal cortex.

Based on data in their preliminary report (Goyer et al. 1991), Goyer and colleagues (1994) published a more extensive article in which they examined nonparametric rather than parametric correlations and in which they used an analysis of covariance to correct for age and sex differences between the personality disorder patients and the healthy control subjects. Although there were some differences in P values, the overall findings were essentially unchanged. Specifically, in the orbital frontal cortex approximately 40mm above the CML, there was still a significant inverse correlation between absolute scores on the Modified Aggression Scale (MAS; Goyer et al. 1994) and rCMRG ($r = .54$, $P = .025$). Compared with that of healthy control subjects, rCMRG in the frontal lobes of the borderline patients was decreased in the transaxial plane approximately 81mm above the CML and increased in the plane approximately 53mm above the CML ($F[1,45] = 8.65$, $P = .005$; and $F[1,45] = 7.68$, $P = .008$, respectively) (Goyer et al. 1994).

Data supporting decreased orbital frontal and prefrontal cortical metabolism in violent behavior have also been reported by Volkow and Tancredi (1987). These investigators used PET to examine regional cerebral blood flow (rCBF) in four psychiatric inpatients with a history of at least three arrests for violent behavior. The ratios of left/right (L/R) temporal and frontal/occipital (F/O) cortex were compared with those of four healthy control subjects. Because of the small numbers, statistical comparisons were not possible. The tabular data were, however, consistent with lowered L/R and F/O ratios in the patients with a history of violent behavior.

Unless one considers the possibility that obsessive-compulsive disorder (OCD) has a strong personality disorder component, we know of no other PET studies in personality disorder patients apart from those of Goyer et al. and Raine et al. Some authors have reported increases in rCMRG in the orbital frontal and prefrontal cortex of patients with OCD compared with non-psychiatrically ill control groups (Baxter et al. 1987, 1988, 1989; Benkelfat et al. 1990; Nordahl et al. 1989; Swedo et al. 1989). However, Martinot et al. (1990b) have reported *decreases* in these regions. OCD has also been studied with SPECT (Machlin et al. 1991; Rubin et al. 1992; Zohar et al. 1989). These and other functional brain imaging studies in OCD have been reviewed by Baxter (1992). While the findings in the prefrontal cortex of the BPD patients may partially overlap with some of the reported OCD findings, the decrease in normalized rCMRG in the higher transaxial plane of the frontal cortex does not. Within the entire group of 17 personality disorder patients (Goyer et al. 1991, 1994), the inverse correlation of trait aggression with rCMRG suggests that a higher rCMRG in the orbital frontal cortex is associated with less aggressive impulse difficulty. The possibility exists that the OCD diagnostic group finding of orbital frontal increases in rCMRG may also be related to symptom inhibition of aggressive impulses.

CONCLUSIONS

The few studies that have used brain imaging have shown that this technique may become a powerful tool in the search for a pathophysiology of borderline and/or schizotypal personality disorders. The results of structural imaging studies seem to indicate that patients with BPD do not have the same parameters as patients with schizophrenia or with delusional depression—that is, borderline patients do not appear to have enlarged ventricles. This finding should, however, be stated with caution because the total number of borderline subjects studied has been quite small and also because there are no known studies that have employed the MRI, a more sensitive instrument. In patients with SPD (either alone or comorbid with other personality or Axis I diagnoses), however, ventricular size is either enlarged (Siever 1991) or appears correlated with global severity of illness (Konicki et al. 1992). Although the results to date are not striking, we suggest that sufficient preliminary data exist to pursue MRI studies in these personality disorders.

As our understanding of imaging becomes more sophisticated, we should, in future studies, examine areas of the brain beyond ventricular size. In addition, there may be fruitful research in exploring sulcal prominence, since there is some evidence that this parameter may now be assessed more validly than was possible just a few years ago. The role of the frontal cortex in BPD may prove to be as interesting as it appears to be in schizophrenia (Weinberger 1987), and perhaps may eventually explain specific disinhibited responses to stress or medication (Gardner and Cowdry 1985).

However, we think that as much potential as there is for structural imaging, the possibilities for functional imaging are greater. The findings for other disorders such as panic—in which no structural abnormalities have been reported, yet functional parameters have been found to be abnormal (Nordahl et al. 1990; Reiman et al. 1984, 1986)—lead us to believe that this area is worthy of concentrated effort in personality disorder patients. The results of the Goyer et al. preliminary report in 1991 and of their more extensive 1994 report indicate strong metabolic correlations to MAS measures of aggression and impulsivity. The reports point to the potential power of this technique in furthering our understanding not only of BPD, but also of the more troubling impulsive behavior found in this disorder. In addition, the development and use of PET with 5-hydroxytryptamine (5-HT) receptor ligands or 5-HT pharmacological probes (Goyer et al. 1993) may throw further light on the relationship of serotonin to some aspects of borderline behavior (see Chapter 2).

Future brain imaging studies should include pharmacological and/or cognitive activation probes during functional brain imaging scans. Imaginative strategies in this area may not only lead to a better clinical understanding of BPD and SPD, but may also provide a jumping-off point for more sophisticated research into the personality disorders.

REFERENCES

Akiskal HS: Subaffective disorders: dysthymic, cyclothymic, and bipolar II disorders in the "borderline" realm. Psychiatr Clin North Am 4:25–46, 1981

American Psychiatric Association: Diagnostic and Statistical Manual of Mental Disorders, 3rd Edition, Revised. Washington, DC, American Psychiatric Association, 1987

Andrulonis PA, Glueck BC, Stroebel CF, et al: Organic brain dysfunction and the borderline syndrome. Psychiatr Clin North Am 4:47–66, 1981

Baxter LR: Neuroimaging studies of obsessive compulsive disorder. Psychiatr Clin North Am 15:871–884, 1992

Baxter LR, Phelps ME, Mazziotta JC, et al: Cerebral metabolic rates for glucose in mood disorders. Arch Gen Psychiatry 42:441–447, 1985

Baxter LR, Phelps ME, Mazziotta JC, et al: Local cerebral glucose metabolic rates in obsessive-compulsive disorder: a comparison with rates in unipolar depression and in normal controls. Arch Gen Psychiatry 44:211–218, 1987

Baxter LR, Schwartz JM, Mazziotta JC, et al: Cerebral glucose metabolic rates in nondepressed patients with obsessive-compulsive disorder. Am J Psychiatry 145:1560–1563, 1988

Baxter LR, Schwartz JM, Phelps ME, et al: Reduction of prefrontal cortex glucose metabolism common to three types of depression. Arch Gen Psychiatry 46:243–250, 1989

Benkelfat C, Nordahl TE, Semple WE, et al: Local cerebral glucose metabolic rates in obsessive-compulsive disorder. Arch Gen Psychiatry 47:840–848, 1990

Braff DL: Impaired speed of information processing in nonmedicated schizotypal patients. Schizophr Bull 7:499–508, 1981

Brown GL, Goodwin FK, Ballenger JC, et al: Aggression in humans: correlates with cerebrospinal fluid amine metabolites. Psychiatry Res 1:131–139, 1979

Brown GL, Ebert MH, Goyer PF, et al: Aggression, suicide, and serotonin: relationships to CSF amine metabolites. Am J Psychiatry 139:741–746, 1982

Buchsbaum MS, Cappelletti J, Ball R, et al: Positron emission tomographic image measurement in schizophrenia and affective disorders. Ann Neurol 15:S157–S165, 1984

Cloninger CR: A systematic method for clinical description and classification of personality variants: a proposal. Arch Gen Psychiatry 44:573–588, 1987

Coccaro EF, Siever LJ, Klar HM, et al: Serotonergic studies in patients with affective and personality disorders: correlates with suicidal and impulsive aggressive behavior. Arch Gen Psychiatry 46:587–599, 1989

Coccaro EF, Gabriel S, Siever LJ: Buspirone challenge: preliminary evidence for a role for central 5-HT$_{1a}$ receptor function in impulsive aggressive behavior in humans. Psychopharmacol Bull 26:393–405, 1990

Coffey CE, Figiel GS, Djang WT, et al: White matter hyperintensity on magnetic resonance imaging: clinical and neuroanatomic correlates in the depressed elderly. J Neuropsychiatry Clin Neurosci 1:135–144, 1989

Cohen RM, Semple WE, Gross M, et al: Dysfunction in a prefrontal substrate of sustained attention in schizophrenia. Life Sci 40:2031–2039, 1987

Cohen RM, Semple WE, Gross M, et al: Evidence for common alterations in cerebral glucose metabolism in major affective disorders and schizophrenia. Neuropsychopharmacology 2:241–254, 1989

Cornelius JR, Soloff PH, Geroge AWA, et al: An evaluation of the significance of selected neuropsychiatric abnormalities in the etiology of borderline personality disorder. Journal of Personality Disorders 3:19–25, 1989

Cowdry RW, Gardner DL: Pharmacotherapy of borderline personality disorder: alprazolam, carbamazepine, trifluoperazine and tranylcypromine. Arch Gen Psychiatry 45:111–119, 1988

Cowdry RW, Pickar D, Davies R: Symptoms and EEG findings in the borderline syndrome. Int J Psychiatry Med 15:201–211, 1985–1986

Dupont RM, Jernigan TL, Gillin JC, et al: Subcortical signal hyperintensities in bipolar patients detected by MRI. Psychiatry Res 21:357–358, 1987

Frances A, Clarkin JF, Gilmore M, et al: Reliability of criteria for borderline personality disorder: a comparison of DSM-III and diagnostic interview for borderline patients. Am J Psychiatry 141:1080–1084, 1984

Garbutt JC, Loosen PT, Tipermas A, et al: The TRH test in patients with borderline personality disorder. Psychiatry Res 9:107–113, 1983

Gardner DL, Cowdry RW: Alprazolam-induced dyscontrol in borderline personality disorder. Am J Psychiatry 142:98–100, 1985

Gardner DL, Lucas PB, Cowdry RW: Soft sign neurological abnormalities in borderline personality disorder and normal control subjects. J Nerv Ment Dis 175:177–180, 1987

Gold LJ, Silk KR: Exploring the borderline personality disorder–major affective disorder interface, in Borderline Personality Disorder: Etiology and Treatment. Edited by Paris J. Washington, DC, American Psychiatric Press, 1993, pp 39–66

Goyer PF, Andreason PJ, Semple WE, et al: PET and personality disorders (abstract). Biol Psychiatry 29 (no 9A):94A, 1991

Goyer PF, Schulz PM, Semple WE, et al: Cerebral glucose metabolism in patients with summer seasonal affective disorder. Neuropsychopharmacology 7:233–240, 1992

Goyer PF, Semple WE, Morris ED, et al: Effects of MK-212 on regional cerebral blood flow in humans (letter). Schizophr Res 9:199, 1993

Goyer PF, Andreason PJ, Semple WE, et al: Positron-emission tomography and personality disorders. Neuropsychopharmacology 10:21–28, 1994

Gunderson JG, Elliott GR: The interface between borderline personality disorder and affective disorder. Am J Psychiatry 142:277–288, 1985

Gunderson JG, Phillips KA: A current view of the interface between borderline personality disorder and depression. Am J Psychiatry 148:967–975, 1991

Gunderson JG, Kolb JE, Austin V: The Diagnostic Interview for Borderline Patients. Am J Psychiatry 138:896–903, 1981

Gunderson JG, Siever LJ, Spauldin E: The search for a schizotype: crossing the border again. Arch Gen Psychiatry 40:15–22, 1983

Gunderson JG, Singer MT: Defining borderline patients: an overview. Am J Psychiatry 132:1–10, 1975

Kety SS, Rosenthal D, Wender PH, et al: Mental illness in the biological and adoptive families of adopted individuals who have become schizophrenic: preliminary report based on psychiatric interviews, in Genetic Research in Psychiatry. Edited by Fieve RR, Rosenthal D, Brill H. Baltimore, MD, John Hopkins University Press, 1975, pp 147–165

Kolb JE, Gunderson JG: Diagnosing borderline patients with a semistructured interview. Arch Gen Psychiatry 37:37–41, 1980

Konicki PE, Shea MT, Fenton WS, et al: Brain structure and severity in borderline disorder. Paper presented at the 145th annual meeting of the American Psychiatric Association, Washington, DC, May 1992

Korzekwa M, Links P, Steiner M: Biological markers in borderline personality disorder: new perspectives. Can J Psychiatry 36 (suppl 1, Feb):1–5, 1993

Lahmeyer HW, Reynolds CF III, Kupfer DJ, et al: Biologic markers in borderline personality disorder: a review. J Clin Psychiatry 50:217–225, 1989

Lidberg L, Tuck JR, Åsberg M, et al: Homicide, suicide and CSF 5-HIAA. Acta Psychiatr Scand 71:230–236, 1985

Linnoila M, Virkkunen M, Scheinin M, et al: Low cerebrospinal fluid 5-hydroxyindoleacetic acid concentration differentiates impulsive from nonimpulsive violent behavior. Life Sci 33:2609–2614, 1983

Loranger AW: Personality Disorder Examination Manual. Yonkers, NY, DV Communications, 1988

Lucas PB, Gardner DL, Cowdry RW, et al: Cerebral structure in borderline personality disorder. Psychiatry Res 27:111–115, 1989

Machlin SR, Harris GJ, Pearlson GD, et al: Elevated medial-frontal cerebral blood flow in obsessive-compulsive patients: a SPECT study. Am J Psychiatry 148:1240–1242, 1991

Markovitz PJ, Calabrese JR, Schulz SC, et al: Fluoxetine in the treatment of borderline and schizotypal personality disorders. Am J Psychiatry 148:1064–1067, 1991

Martinot JL, Hardy P, Feline A, et al: Left prefrontal glucose hypometabolism in the depressed state: a confirmation. Am J Psychiatry 147:1313–1317, 1990a

Martinot JL, Allilaire JF, Mazoyer BM, et al: Obsessive-compulsive disorder: a clinical, neuropsychological, and positron emission tomography study. Acta Psychiatr Scand 82:233–242, 1990b

McNamara E, Reynolds CF III, Soloff PH, et al: EEG sleep evaluation of depression in borderline patients. Am J Psychiatry 141:182–186, 1984

Nordahl TE, Benkelfat C, Semple WE, et al: Cerebral glucose metabolic rates in obsessive compulsive disorder. Neuropsychopharmacology 2:23–28, 1989

Nordahl TE, Semple WE, Gross M, et al: Cerebral glucose metabolic differences in patients with panic disorder. Neuropsychopharmacology 3:261–272, 1990

Overall JE, Gorham DR: The Brief Psychiatric Rating Scale. Psychol Rep 10:799–812, 1962

Parnas J, Teasdale TW: A matched-paired comparison of treated versus untreated schizophrenia spectrum cases: a high-risk population study. Acta Psychiatr Scand 75:44–50, 1987

Raine A, Buchsbaum MS, Stanley J, et al: Selective reductions in prefrontal glucose metabolism in murderers assessed with positron emission tomography. Psychophysiology 29 (suppl 4A):S–58, 1992

Reiman EM, Raichle ME, Butler FK, et al: A focal brain abnormality in panic disorder, a severe form of anxiety. Nature 310:683–685, 1984

Reiman EM, Raichle ME, Robins E, et al: The application of positron emission tomography to the study of panic disorder. Am J Psychiatry 143:469–477, 1986

Roy A, Linnoila M: Suicidal behavior, impulsiveness and serotonin. Acta Psychiatry Scand 78:529–535, 1988

Rubin RT, Villanueva-Meyer J, Ananth J, et al: Regional ^{133}Xe cerebral blood flow and cerebral ^{99m}HMPAO uptake in unmedicated obsessive-compulsive disorder patients and matched normal control subjects: determination by high-resolution single-photon emission computed tomography. Arch Gen Psychiatry 49:695–702, 1992

Schulz SC, Koller MM, Kishore PR, et al: Ventricular enlargement in teenage patients with schizophrenia spectrum disorder. Am J Psychiatry 140:1592–1595, 1983

Semple WE, Goyer PF, McCormick R, et al: Preliminary report: brain blood flow using PET in patients with posttraumatic stress disorder and substance-abuse histories. Biol Psychiatry 34:115–118, 1993

Siever LJ: The biology of the boundaries of schizophrenia, in Advances in Neuropsychiatry and Psychopharmacology, Vol 1: Schizophrenia Research. Edited by Tamminga CA, Schulz SC. New York, Raven, 1991, pp 181–191

Siever LJ, Davis KL: A psychobiological perspective on the personality disorders. Am J Psychiatry 148:1647–1658, 1991

Siever LJ, Coursey RD, Alterman IS, et al: Impaired smooth pursuit eye movement: a vulnerability marker for schizotypal personality disorder in a normal volunteer population. Am J Psychiatry 141:1560–1566, 1984

Siever LJ, Coccaro EF, Zemishlany Z, et al: Psychobiology of personality disorders: pharmacologic implications. Psychopharmacol Bull 23:333–336, 1987

Siever LJ, Amin F, Coccaro EF, et al: Plasma homovanillic acid in schizotypal personality disorder patients and controls. Am J Psychiatry 148:1246–1248, 1991

Silk KR, Feinberg M, Lohr NE, et al: Sleep EEG versus DST in borderlines with melancholia. Paper presented at the 138th annual meeting of the American Psychiatric Association, Dallas, TX, May 1985

Soloff PH, Ulrich RF: Diagnostic interview for borderline patients: a replication study. Arch Gen Psychiatry 38:686–692, 1981

Spitzer RL, Endicott J: Schedule for Affective Disorders and Schizophrenia (Lifetime Version), 3rd Edition. New York, New York State Psychiatric Institute, 1978

Spitzer RL, Endicott J, Gibbon M: Crossing the border into borderline personality and borderline schizophrenia: the development of criteria. Arch Gen Psychiatry 36:17–24, 1979

Sternbach HA, Fleming J, Extein I, et al: The dexamethasone suppression and thyrotropin-releasing hormone tests in depressed borderline patients. Psychoneuroendocrinology 8:459–462, 1983

Stone MH: Contemporary shift of the borderline concept from a sub-schizophrenic disorder to a subaffective disorder. Psychiatr Clin North Am 2:577–594, 1979

Swedo SE, Schapiro MB, Grady CL, et al: Cerebral glucose metabolism in childhood-onset obsessive-compulsive disorder. Arch Gen Psychiatry 46:518–523, 1989

Targum SD, Rosen LN, DeLisi LE, et al: Cerebral ventricular size in major depressive disorder: association with delusional symptoms. Biol Psychiatry 18:329–336, 1983

Virkkunen M, Nuutila A, Goodwin FK, et al: Cerebrospinal fluid monoamine metabolite levels in male arsonists. Arch Gen Psychiatry 44:241–247, 1987

Volkow ND, Tancredi L: Neural substrates of violent behavior: a preliminary study with positron emission tomography. Br J Psychiatry 151:668–673, 1987

Weinberger DR: Implications of normal brain development for the pathogenesis of schizophrenia. Arch Gen Psychiatry 44:660–669, 1987

Weinberger DR, Berman KF, Zec RF: Physiologic dysfunction of dorsolateral prefrontal cortex in schizophrenia, I: regional cerebral blood flow (CBF) evidence. Arch Gen Psychiatry 43:114–124, 1986

Zametkin AJ, Nordahl TE, Gross M, et al: Cerebral glucose metabolism in adults with hyperactivity of childhood onset. N Eng J Med 323:1361–1366, 1990

Zanarini MC, Gunderson JG, Frankenburg FR, et al: The revised diagnostic interview for borderlines: discriminating BPD from other Axis II disorders. Journal of Personality Disorders 3:10–18, 1989

Zohar J, Insel TR, Berman KF, et al: Anxiety and cerebral blood flow during behavioral challenge: dissociation of central from peripheral and subjective measures. Arch Gen Psychiatry 46:505–510, 1989

Chapter 7

Neuropsychological Testing Results in Borderline Personality Disorder

Kathleen M. O'Leary, M.S.W.
Rex William Cowdry, M.D.

Among the prominent characteristics of borderline personality disorder (BPD) described in the classic literature are a number of pathological features with strong cognitive components: the use of projection and splitting, distorted part-object representations of other individuals, selective forgetting of past experiences, difficulty differentiating present experiences from expectations based upon the past, and difficulties in binding anxiety through thought rather than relieving it through action. Clinicians who work extensively with individuals with BPD experience concrete examples of these cognitive shortcomings in their day-to-day encounters with these patients. They forget appointments, say they cannot recall the faces of significant people in their lives, misperceive situations, overreact to minor events, fail to anticipate the consequences of their actions, seem to make only slow progress in psychotherapy and, more generally, appear unable to learn from experience.

Until recently, these cognitive phenomena have not been closely examined through quantitative research methods. There are several reasons for the delay. First, it has been assumed that

---

The authors would like to thank James Gold, Ph.D., of the National Institute of Mental Health Clinical Research Services Branch for his generous assistance in the preparation of this chapter.

the cognitive style, memory lapses, and misperceptions that these patients display are psychodynamically defensive in origin—they are born of the need to ward off intolerable feelings, memories, or conflicts. In addition, the cognitive stylistic features of borderline patients, such as poor logic, confused thinking, and distortions, have been recently deemphasized in the continuing effort to distinguish the diagnostic criteria for BPD from those for schizotypal personality disorder (Kroll 1988). Finally, these phenomena have not been extensively studied from a neuropsychological perspective because of the long-standing belief that borderline patients appear to be "normal" on structured psychological tests. This latter belief derives from the literature, which reportedly shows a pattern of normal, unremarkable functioning on the Wechsler Adult Intelligence Scale (WAIS) with severe psychopathology only on unstructured projective tests, such as the Rorschach. This belief also fits with clinical impressions that the BPD population shows a normal distribution of intelligence, with many borderline individuals functioning well in structured work situations.

Several recent, small-scale studies suggest that the above assumptions—that borderline individuals perform normally on structured standardized tests and that defensive operations of the ego are the sole source of cognitive distortions and lapses—need to be reexamined. Three studies will be described that have found that borderline patients experience difficulties on structured neuropsychological tests that assess nonconflictual, nonaffect-laden learning. While these studies are preliminary and further research is needed, the three studies uncovered strikingly similar findings of impairment in the areas of memory and visuospatial processing in the borderline patients compared with healthy control subjects.

In this chapter we summarize other evidence that justifies consideration of a neurological or organic basis for some of the symptomatology associated with BPD. These findings do not necessarily refute the more traditional psychodynamically based explanations; rather, they may stand alongside those explanations and broaden our understanding of this complex phenomenon known as BPD. In the following sections we briefly describe the relevant neurological studies, raise the question of the role of attention deficits in the disorder, and explore other clinical evidence for an organic component. We also examine the source of the long-held "disturbed Rorschach–intact WAIS" belief and present some of the new data together with a discussion of their meanings and clinical implications.

INDICATIONS OF ORGANIC IMPAIRMENT

Neurological Studies

A number of small-scale studies have demonstrated findings suggestive of neurological impairment in BPD. In their study of borderline adolescents, Andrulonis et al. (1981) found that 14% had a history of brain trauma, seizures, or encephalitis. There have been findings of an increased incidence of nonspecific electroencephalogram (EEG) abnormalities in borderline patients compared with patients with major depression (Cowdry et al. 1985–1986) and with patients with dysthymia (Snyder and Pitts 1984), but the abnormalities found in these two studies were different from each other (an excess of slow-wave activity in one case and an excess of fast activity in the other). Borderline patients also showed an increased incidence of neurological soft sign abnormalities when compared with healthy control subjects (Gardner et al. 1987). However, Cornelius and colleagues (1986) found no increased incidence of EEG abnormalities in borderline patients compared with patients with other personality disorders, and there has been no evidence of focal lesions or ventricular enlargement on computed tomography (CT) imaging studies (Lucas et al. 1989; Snyder et al. 1983). Although the positive studies suggest the possibility of subtle organic dysfunction in some individuals with BPD, it appears that the abnormalities are both nonspecific and nonfocal, and may only affect a subgroup of borderline patients. Neurological dysfunction in the borderline patient is reviewed and discussed in more detail in Chapters 8 and 9. Chapter 6 presents a thorough review of neuroimaging studies and a discussion of their implications for future research in BPD.

Attention Disorders

Another subgroup of borderline patients who may demonstrate specific cognitive impairment are those with a prior history of learning disabilities or attention-deficit hyperactivity disorder (ADHD). Increased incidence of attention disorders or learning disabilities in BPD has been theorized (Christman 1984) and described (Andrulonis et al. 1981, 1982; Cohen et al. 1983), but methodologically rigorous studies with comparison groups have not yet been done. In longitudinal studies of children with attention disorders, the literature has described borderline-like outcomes (Hartocollis 1968) as well as outcomes that may be phenomenologically similar to BPD, such as emotionally unstable character disorder (Quitkin and Klein 1969), labile personality (Wood et al. 1976), and impulsive personality (Weiss 1985). Larger and more recent longitudinal studies of children with ADHD have reported a significant incidence only of antisocial personality disorder (Gittelman et al. 1985; Mannuzza et al. 1989, 1991). However, no systematic method was used to assess for the presence of other personality disorders, and children with ADHD plus primary aggressive behavior/conduct disorder, psychosis, borderline psychosis, or neurological dysfunction were excluded from these longitudinal studies. As Lie (1992) points out in his review, those exclusions could rule out borderline outcomes. Studies of adult ADHD–residual type (ADHD-RT) (Amado and Lustman 1982; Wender et al. 1981, 1985) have also ruled out subjects with BPD. Nonetheless, characteristics of ADHD-RT—particularly the affective lability, impulsivity, and occasional rage—are strikingly similar to diagnostic criteria for BPD. This is not to suggest that ADHD-RT and BPD are the same disorder. Further research will be needed to determine whether there is a distinguishable subgroup of borderline patients characterized by a history of ADHD or learning disability, and whether this group in particular demonstrates the expected neuropsychological test abnormalities.

Clinical Indications

The clinical evidence for possible organic impairment in BPD is anecdotal and nonspecific but may help researchers identify neuropsychological functions of particular interest. The general cognitive style shows "a tendency toward global perceptions with a loss of attention to detail, distortion of the meaning of an event, patterns of confusion and spotty amnesias" (Kroll 1988, p. 71). Borderline patients exhibit different types of attentional difficulties: at times they miss details and facts and at other times they focus exclusively on one small aspect of a situation and then miss the *gestalt*—the context. They show memory difficulties of various types. They cannot remember what they did yesterday, or last week, or what they said in their last therapy session. They cannot remember their positive experiences. And, of course, they tend to have memory lapses surrounding traumatic events.

There are several explanations for these apparent difficulties. The classic explanation is that these lapses serve a defensive function, and that they are motivated by unconscious conflicts. These difficulties could also be partially accounted for by state-dependent learning. We know that retention and retrieval of information are influenced by the mood state in which the material is learned (Eich 1980; Eich et al. 1975; Lewinsohn and Rosenbaum 1987), and borderline patients have very labile mood states. In addition, memory problems may arise from severe cases of state-dependent learning and recall, such as during dissociative periods or—in the extreme—in multiple personality disorder.

Similar questions of etiology and meaning occur with the other cognitive difficulties. Borderline patients have difficulty interpreting complex situations and establishing causal connections (Westen et al. 1990a). They seem unable to learn from their mistakes by applying past learning to present situations. As Westen et al. (1990b) point out, it is not sufficient to attribute this lack of appreciation/integration of past experience to an arrested emotional development, as if object relations were a monolithic developmental process or structure. These issues lead one to consider the dimensions of specific problems in learning, recall, or abstract thinking. Borderline patients appear intolerant of ambiguity. Although splitting clearly serves an important psychological defensive function (Gabbard 1989; Kernberg 1975), it could also reflect a neurological disturbance in information processing (Muller 1992). If someone is perceptually confused or impaired, perhaps simple categorization that allows only either/or, black/white decisions is the cognitive path of least resistance.

EVIDENCE FROM PSYCHOLOGICAL TESTING

Past Studies

"Disturbed Rorschach–Intact WAIS" Pattern

For several decades, the precept "disturbed Rorschach–intact WAIS" has been the main assumption regarding the functioning of borderline patients on psychological tests. According to this paradigm, borderline patients perform well on structured tests such as the WAIS, but on projective tests such as the Rorschach they reveal psychotic thought patterns that at times appear even more disturbed than the responses given by schizophrenic patients. However, there has not been a current, methodologically rigorous study to test this premise. Furthermore, careful examination of the history of this hypothesis suggests that it is based on an overinterpretation of seminal studies of patients who were most likely more schizotypal than borderline.

The Rorschach

The origin of the belief in borderline patients' extremely psychotic Rorschach responses began with Rorschach himself. He first mentioned in passing patients with "latent schizophrenia" who may look more disturbed on his test than patients with "manifest schizophrenia" (Rorschach 1921, revised 1942, 1975). The subsequent classic study by Rapaport and colleagues (Rapaport et al. 1945–1946, revised 1968) examined two groups of "preschizophrenics" with the Rorschach. One group was described as "overideational," or loose, and the other as "coarctated," or constricted. It has been assumed that these "overideational preschizophrenics," with their floridly emotional and psychopathological responses, were borderline.

However, this work by Rapaport et al. was done decades before the DSM-III (American Psychiatric Association 1980) formulation of borderline personality disorder. Holt, the editor of the later edition of Rapaport et al.'s *Diagnostic Psychological Testing* (1968), M. H. Stone, who examined the early conceptualization of the disorder (1980), and Widiger, in his thorough review article (1982), all seem to agree that the patients described by Rapaport and colleagues were, in all likelihood, not borderline. And, as Widiger details, the subsequent commonly cited sources of the belief that borderline subjects decompensate to an extreme degree on the Rorschach (McCully 1962; Mercer and Wright 1950; Schafer 1948, 1954; H. K. Stone and Dellis 1960; Weiner 1966; Zucker 1952) are problematic when viewed by today's standards of diagnosis, methodology, and interpretation.

This is not to challenge the idea that borderline patients display characteristic psychopathology on the Rorschach. According to recent studies, borderline patients do indeed exhibit characteristic responses on the Rorschach. However, Singer and Larson's (1981) often-quoted findings that differentiated borderline patients from healthy, neurotic, and schizophrenic subjects are questionable because "the majority of our sample would have met the schizotypal criteria" (Singer and Larson 1981, p. 695). Exner (1986) presents the most thorough recent study of borderline performance on the Rorschach. He found that the Rorschachs of borderline patients differed significantly from those of schizotypal and schizophrenic patients. The schizotypal patients' Rorschachs looked more like those of the schizophrenic patients, whereas the borderline patients exhibited a distinctive form of personality disorganization manifested by affect modulation problems coupled with impairment in control and increased egocentricity. Borderline patients showed less cognitive slippage and less distortion than the other groups. Other researchers who have recently examined the Rorschach in terms of defensive patterns (Lerner 1990), ego functioning (Berg 1990), or object relations (Stuart et al. 1990) have also noted specific findings that distinguish borderline patients from other diagnostic groups, but these findings are not those suggested by the original term "disturbed Rorschach."

The WAIS

It is reasonable to assume that borderline subjects would produce WAIS results within normal limits. They do not exhibit gross impairment on mental status examination. Many individuals with this disorder function well in intellectually demanding jobs. Again, however, many of the studies commonly cited as supportive of this belief (Rapaport et al. 1945–1946/1968) were based on a different, pre-DSM-III concept of the disorder, and many studies lacked a comparison group (H. K. Stone and Dellis 1960). Some studies cited to support the entire "disturbed Rorschach–intact WAIS" equation present only Rorschach material (Blatt and Ritzler 1974; Edell 1987; Fisher 1955; McCully 1962; Singer and Larson 1981; Wilson 1985; Zucker 1952); others are single-case studies (Carr and Goldstein 1981; Mercer and Wright 1950; Shapiro 1954/1960); and still others simply restate the hypothesis (Forer 1950; Gunderson and Singer 1975; Schafer 1954; Singer 1977; Weiner 1966). Gruenewald (1970) administered a thorough battery, including the WAIS and the Rorschach, to 10 of Grinker et al.'s (1968) borderline patients. She presents no data, but found that the test battery alone was not diagnostic in 7 out of 10 cases. Finally, those who have concluded that functioning is "intact" on the WAIS examined the WAIS solely for thought disorder (Armstrong et al. 1986; Carr et al. 1979; Hymowitz et al. 1983; Patrick and Wolfe 1983).

The only firm conclusions that can be drawn from these studies are that the Rorschach appears useful for distinguishing individuals with BPD from some other diagnostic groups, and that borderline individuals do not display thought disorder on the WAIS. However, the Rorschach comparison studies need to be extended to affective disorders and other personality disorders. The WAIS conclusion, moreover, may not be specific to BPD: we would suspect that many psychiatrically disordered groups would not display thought disorder on the WAIS. But the point that is often overlooked is that the WAIS was not designed to assess thought disorder. Thus, the phrase "adequate WAIS functioning" has divergent meanings when it is used to assess the presence of thought disorder versus cognitive neuropsychological functioning.

Recent Studies

In order to explore further the question of cognitive functioning in borderline patients, we next review the results of four recent studies of neuropsychological testing of borderline subjects. Cornelius et al. (1989) administered a full neuropsychological battery including the WAIS to 24 borderline subjects. They found no deficits specific to borderline patients on the WAIS or any other tests; however, they used historical norms rather than a comparison group. Three other groups of researchers, including our own, have compared borderline subjects with healthy control subjects and found deficits among the borderline subjects on the same subtest of the Wechsler Adult Intelligence Scale—Revised (WAIS-R; Wechsler 1981)—the Digit Symbol—as well as in the areas of visuospatial skills and memory (Carpenter et al. 1993; Judd and Ruff 1993; O'Leary et al. 1991). In addition, Burgess (1990) administered to both borderline and control subjects a brief cognitive exam that combined elements from the mental status exam with items similar to those on a neurological soft signs exam. Although Burgess found significant between-group differences in mental arithmetic, memory, and motor skills, he did not control for IQ or other possibly significant intervening variables.

The main findings that discriminated the borderline patients from the control subjects in the four studies mentioned directly above are presented in Table 7–1 and discussed below. Following a discussion of the results, we summarize those tests that showed no significant difference between borderline and control subjects. We then discuss possible contributory factors that may have affected the test results.

New WAIS Findings

The Digit Symbol is a timed coding test that requires the subject to look at a line of nonsense symbols paired with numbers and to write the correct corresponding symbol below under a sequence of numbers. It is considered a test of attention, visuomotor coordination, and perceptual organization (Lezak 1983). As shown in Table 7–1, we found a significant difference only on the Digit

Table 7-1. Categories showing significant neuropsychological test findings in borderline patients (versus control subjects)

		Visuospatial skills			Memory		
Study	WAIS-R subtests	Copy a design	Attention/ perception/ disembedding	Simple visual	Complex visual	Simple verbal	Complex verbal
Burgess (1990)	NA	NA	NA	NA	NA	Three Word Pairs*	NA
Carpenter et al. (1993)	Digit Symbol* Block Design* Vocabulary	Rey-Osterrieth* (Block Design)	Trails A and B* (Block Design) (Digit Symbol) Continuous Performance Task	WMS-R Visual Reproduction*	Rey-Osterrieth*	NA	WMS-R Logical Memory
Judd and Ruff (1993)	Digit Symbol* Block Design Vocabulary Information Digit Span Comprehension Similarities Picture Completion	Rey-Osterrieth*	Ruff Figural Fluency* Corsi/Block Span* (Digit Symbol*)	NA	(Rey-Osterrieth*) (Corsi/Block Span*)	Selective Reminding Test	WMS-R Logical Memory*

Study	Wechsler	Rey-Osterrieth	Embedded Figures/Other	WMS-R Visual Reproduction	Rey-Osterrieth*	WMS-R Associate Learning	WMS-R Logical Memory*
O'Leary et al. (1991)	Digit Symbol* Block Design Vocabulary Information Digit Span Arithmetic Comprehension Similarities Picture Completion Picture Arrangement Object Assembly	Rey-Osterrieth	Embedded Figures* Road-Map* Corsi/Block Span* Visual Search		(Embedded Figures*) (Corsi/Block Span*)		

Note. NA = not administered. WMS-R = Wechsler Memory Scale—Revised (Wechsler 1987). Parentheses indicate that the test has also been listed for that study in a prior category. The performance of the borderline patients was worse than that of the control subjects in all cases. *$P < .05$.

Symbol subtest when 16 borderline patients were compared with 16 control subjects on the full WAIS-R with its 11 subtests (O'Leary et al. 1991). There was a significant difference between our two groups in Performance IQ as well, but this was attributable to the Digit Symbol, since there were no significant differences on any other subtests. Judd and Ruff (1993) also found a significant difference only on the Digit Symbol when they compared 25 borderline and matched archival healthy control subjects on 8 of the 11 WAIS-R subtests. Carpenter et al. (1993) found significant deficits on the Digit Symbol and on the Block Design when they compared 17 borderline and control subjects on three of the WAIS-R subtests. The Block Design requires timed three-dimensional replication of two-dimensional designs, and measures problem solving, visuomotor coordination, and visuospatial organization (Lezak 1983). In each of these cases, borderline performance was significantly worse than that of control subjects.

While it is believed that the Digit Symbol is more sensitive to minimal brain damage than are other WAIS subtests (Hirschenfang 1960) and may measure information-processing capacity (Royer 1971), it is difficult to derive meaning from this single finding without considering it within the context of other cognitive performance findings described below.

Visuospatial Findings

All three studies administered the Rey-Osterrieth (Lezak 1983; Osterrieth 1944) and found significant differences between borderline patients and healthy control subjects. Two of the three studies administered the same block memory test—known as either the Block Span or the Corsi Blocks (Milner 1971)—and found significant differences between groups. Each study also administered other visuospatial tests and found significant differences between groups. In all cases, borderline performance was significantly worse than that of control subjects.

The Rey-Osterrieth requires the subject to copy and then draw from memory a complex geometric figure. It assesses visuospatial organization, visual memory, and visuomotor skills. The first recall is after a brief intervening task and the second is after 45–50 minutes. Judd and Ruff (1993) found the performance of the borderline patients to be significantly impaired on both the copy and the combined recall portions of this test; our group found borderline impairment not on the copy but on both recall portions; and Carpenter and colleagues' (1993) study found impairment on recall but not copy.

The Corsi Blocks/Block Span is the visual analog to the WAIS-R Digit Span subtest. It requires subjects to remember and point out increasingly long patterns of three-dimensional blocks on a board. It tests visual attention, visuospatial organization, and short-term visual memory. Our group required subjects to recall immediately the patterns forward and backward, and we found significant impairment among the borderline subjects on both forward and backward recall. Judd and Ruff (1993) required recall after a 20-second distractor task and found impairment after this brief delay as well.

Each study also found additional deficits on visuospatial tasks that were not administered by the other studies. Our group found borderline impairment on the Embedded Figures Test (Witkin et al. 1971) and significantly slower borderline performance on the Road-Map Test of Direction Sense (Money 1976). The Embedded Figures Test requires subjects to remember a simple geometric shape that is shown and removed, and then to use visual discrimination and filtering to identify that shape within a more complex one. The Road-Map Test assesses spatial orientation and visual discrimination by requiring the subject to describe turns in the path the examiner is tracing among a grid of lines. Judd and Ruff (1993) found significantly worse borderline performance on the Ruff Figural Fluency Test (Ruff et al. 1987), which measures visual fluency, planning, and organization by asking subjects to make as many different designs as possible within a time period by connecting dots with lines. Carpenter et al. (1993) found significantly worse borderline performance on the Visual Reproduction (immediate and delayed) subtest of the Wechsler Memory Scale—Revised (WMS-R; Wechsler 1987) and on the Trail Making Test A and B (Lezak 1983; Reitan 1971). The Visual Reproduction subtest requires the subject to draw from memory some fairly simple geometric designs. Our study found no group differences on this test with the original, unrevised version of the WMS. The Trail Making Test is a timed task requiring the subject to first connect consecutively numbered circles with lines, and then to connect numbered and lettered circles by alternating between the two sequences. It assesses visual attention, visual conceptual skills, and visuomotor tracking.

Two factors must be considered with these findings. One is graphomotor skills, which affect performance on the Digit Symbol subtest, the Rey-Osterrieth copy, the Ruff Figural Fluency Test, and the Trail Making Test. Judd and Ruff (1993) concluded that a motor problem did not explain the visuospatial results because their study showed no significant group differences on either the Grooved Pegboard Test (Lezak 1983) or the Finger Tapping Test (Reitan and Davison 1974). Our group also concluded that the visuospatial group differences were not due to a motor problem because, of the four WAIS-R performance tests with a motor component (Object Assembly, Block Design, Picture Arrangement, and Digit Symbol), only the Digit Symbol showed a significant difference between borderline and control subjects. It seems unlikely that motor tasks requiring the use of a pen or pencil are the specific culprit, but the question of visuomotor impairment requires further study.

The other factor relates to visual attention. Carpenter et al.'s (1993) study was the only protocol that administered a continuous performance task. This study found no significant group differences. Our study administered the Visual Search and Neglect Test, an attentional test described in our report (O'Leary et al. 1991), and Judd and Ruff (1993) administered the 2 and 7 Test of Selection and Sustained Attention (R. M. Ruff, "San Diego Neuropsychological Battery" [unpublished manuscript], University of California, San Diego, 1985). Both tests require high attention, sustained motivation, and graphomotor skill; neither study found group differences. Anxiety, particularly as reflected on timed tasks, may also affect attention. We examined all tests in which speed of response is a factor and, in our battery, the borderline performance was significantly worse in only two out of seven timed tests. Of the remaining tests in which group differences were nonsignificant, borderline performance was slightly better on one and slightly worse on four. Of the tests in which time was derived as a separate score, the patients were faster on one, and the control subjects on two. The only significant (poorer performance) difference was on the Road-Map Test.

Although there are some areas of discrepancy in the visuospatial tests among the studies, the similarity of the findings is striking. All three studies found impairment on the WAIS-R Digit Symbol, all three found deficits on one or both portions of the Rey-Osterrieth, and both studies that administered the Corsi Blocks/Block Span found deficits.

When we examine these findings as a group, several working hypotheses appear:

1. Borderline individuals may have visuospatial deficits—possibly consisting of problems in attending to or perceiving complex visual arrays (i.e., processing new visual information).
2. Borderline individuals may have a particular problem with visual filtering and discrimination (i.e., filtering out extraneous stimuli and selecting relevant visual details from a complex field). Almost all of the tests that were abnormal—with the possible exception of the WMS Visual Reproduction—depend on this skill.
3. Borderline individuals may have difficulties in recalling visual arrays, as seen in the Rey-Osterrieth recall, the WMS Visual Reproduction, and the Corsi Blocks/Block Span.

Memory Findings

All three groups examined both visual and auditory memory in the borderline and control subjects. Although the findings are suggestive of a memory deficit, they are not uniform across studies.

As described previously, there appear to be differences between borderline patients and control subjects in visual memory. There is strong agreement among the three studies regarding borderline impairment on a fairly complex visual memory task—the Rey-Osterrieth—but disagreement in findings on the more simple visual memory task—the WMS Visual Reproduction. Other visual memory tasks on which patients appeared impaired—the Embedded Figures and the Corsi Blocks/Block Span—have a fair degree of complexity.

There is partial agreement among the three studies regarding verbal memory deficits. The issue of complexity as a factor in verbal recall is unclear. Burgess (1990) reported borderline deficits when he compared patients with healthy subjects on a simple verbal memory task—the Delayed Memory of Three Word Pairs (Strub and Black 1987)—as part of his brief cognitive exam. In an extension of this approach, Burgess (1991) found that borderline subjects performed worse than depressed subjects on this same memory test. Population and methodological characteristics that distinguished his subjects from those in the three other studies we are comparing in this chapter are discussed below and listed in Table 7–2.

We found no impairment on the simple verbal memory test—the WMS Associate Learning subtest of recalling word-pair lists. The more complex WMS Logical Memory subtest requires a subject to recall immediately, and then again after 40–50 minutes, details of two stories of upsetting events that the subject has heard read aloud. While Carpenter et al.'s (1993) patients showed no impairment on this task with the revised WMS (Wechsler 1987), both our study and Judd and Ruff's (1993) study found significant impairment on delayed story recall in the borderline patients with the original WMS (Wechsler and C. P. Stone 1945). We also found impairment on immediate story recall. After administration of the delayed-recall portion, our examiner administered a "cues" section, with prompting questions such as "Do you remember where the robbery took place?" With cueing, the borderline group remembered significantly more additional story elements. When the cued responses are added into the score, borderline performance approached—yet did not quite equal—control performance. This improvement with cueing leads to the speculation that the memory problems experienced by borderline individuals may arise from difficulties in retrieving learned material, rather than from the original encoding process.

The results from the memory testing yield the following hypotheses:

Table 7–2. Methodology and characteristics of borderline patients in neuropsychological studies

	Burgess (1990)	Carpenter et al. (1993)	Judd and Ruff (1993)	O'Leary et al. (1991)
Diagnosis				
DSM-III-R	X	X		X
DSM-III			X	
Diagnostic method				
Interview	X	X		
Interview and DIB			X	X
Current Axis I included	No	Yes	No	Yes
Number of patients	18	17	25	16
Gender	33% F	100% F	80% F	81% F
Setting	Outpatient—acute	Inpatient—long-term	Outpatient—nonacute	Inpatient—for research
Medication status				
Medication free for longer than 2 weeks			X	X
Taking medications	Not available	X		
Substance abuse				
No current; some prior		X	X	X
No drug use for less than 1 week (alcohol unspecified)	X			
IQ assessed	No	Yes	Yes	Yes
Attention assessed	No	Yes	Yes	Yes
Psychomotor skill assessed	No	Yes	Yes	Yes

Note. DIB = Diagnostic Interview for Borderlines (Gunderson et al. 1981).

1. Borderline individuals may have a problem in recalling both visual and verbal material.
2. This memory problem may be more pronounced with complex material.
3. The memory problem may consist of impairment in initial learning and/or retrieval of learned material and may be at least partially correctable by cueing.

Other Test Findings

It should be emphasized that the borderline patients' scores on most tests in each battery showed no significant difference from those of the control subjects. As noted, there was no impairment evident in our borderline subjects on 10 of the 11 WAIS-R subtests. There were no differences in verbal skills between borderline and control subjects. Three studies administered the Wisconsin Card Sorting Test (Heaton 1981), and there were no significant differences between borderline and control subjects on this test of problem solving and adaptability. Borderline patients demonstrated no problems in reasoning on the card sort or on the WAIS-R.

Although we did find poor results among the borderline subjects on some visuospatial tests, there were a number of tasks in which the borderline performance was equal to that of the healthy comparison group. Therefore, borderline subjects do not have an "across-the-board visuospatial deficit." We did not detect any problems among subjects with BPD in elaborating an incomplete drawing on the Street Gestalt Completion Test (Street 1931) or in organizing part elements into a whole on the WAIS-R Object Assembly subtest. In addition, despite anecdotal stories relating to borderline patients' difficulties in remembering the faces of family members, therapists, and so forth, our borderline group showed no impairment on the Facial Memory Test (O'Leary et al. 1991), a pilot test in our battery. However, this test assesses recognition memory rather than the true "evocative memory"—the ability to summon images from within—that is classically reported to be deficient in BPD (Adler and Buie 1979).

Auditory processing problems did not appear to explain verbal memory deficits, since there were no group differences that we found on the Seashore Test of Tonal Memory (Seashore et al. 1960) or that we and Judd and Ruff (1993) found on the Seashore Rhythm Test (Seashore et al. 1960). Deliberately learned material versus incidentally learned material does not appear to explain the borderline deficit. Our study devised two specific tests of incidental memory: the above-described Facial Memory Test and a Verbal Incidental Learning Test (O'Leary et al. 1991). Both subject groups performed equally well. The memory tests on which the borderline subjects appeared impaired included both deliberately learned (e.g., WMS Logical Memory, Embedded Figures) and incidentally learned (e.g., Rey-Osterrieth) tasks.

FACTORS AFFECTING BORDERLINE TEST PERFORMANCE

Table 7–2 examines the important patient characteristics across four studies. All four studies had small cohorts (Burgess [1990]: BPD = 18, Control = 14; Carpenter et al. [1993]: BPD = 17, Control = 17; Judd and Ruff [1993]: BPD = 25, Control = 25; O'Leary et al. [1991]: BPD = 16, Control = 16), yet there were important differences among the populations.

It appears that Carpenter et al.'s (1993) inpatient borderline subjects and possibly Burgess's (1990) outpatients were more severely disturbed than the other two groups. Carpenter et al.'s patients were in a long-term private hospital and Burgess's patients had presented for acute psychiatric hospital assessment. Our borderline group had been functioning as outpatients and entered the hospital in a nonacute phase for research studies. Judd and Ruff's (1993) borderline patients were in ongoing outpatient treatment. Carpenter et al.'s patient group was also taking medication. Burgess provides no medication information. These factors—severity of illness, acuteness, and medication treatment—may explain the impaired performance of these borderline groups on simpler tasks (i.e., WMS Visual Reproduction, Burgess's Delayed Memory of Three Word Pairs) on which the other groups showed no differences.

We examined the possible role of major depression and history of alcohol abuse within the borderline group by comparing test result scores of the patients comorbid for each of these characteristics with the scores of those patients without the characteristic. Although neither current major depression nor a history of alcohol abuse was significantly associated with lower performance on any of the items that discriminated BPD patients from control subjects in our own study, this does not represent conclusive evidence that these factors do not affect test performance.

It is difficult to assess Burgess's 1990 study in relation to the others, primarily due to the gender difference. With a predominantly male population, there may have been much higher rates of ADHD-RT and substance abuse among these subjects, and the lack of measures assessing IQ, attention, and psychomotor skill impair our ability to interpret his findings. Even the larger, later study (Burgess 1991) suffers from these problems, and we have no gender information on the subjects in this study.

INTERPRETATION AND CLINICAL MEANING

These recent studies do lend some support to the earlier supposition that borderline patients appear normal on many structured tests. As a population they may show no obvious problems in verbal skills or reasoning on neuropsychological tests. The impairments in the areas of visuospatial skills and memory may not be readily apparent without detailed testing and comparison with appropriate control subjects. The observed cognitive impairments are not severe. The majority of patients tested with our battery would not have been individually assessed as "grossly impaired." The impairments are evident only when the subjects as a group are compared with a matched, healthy-subject group. It is only then that we can see that the borderline patients' visuospatial skills and memory are not what would be expected considering their IQ, education, and level of other neuropsychological functioning.

Nonetheless, it must be concluded that these deficits are quite real based on our work, as well as that of Carpenter et al. (1993) and Judd and Ruff (1993). Deficits in visuospatial skills and memory definitely were seen in structured testing situations. The test batteries consisted primarily of standardized measures that were not affect-laden and not designed to arouse issues particular to this disorder.

Deficits were evident in only some areas of visuospatial functioning. We interpreted these findings as indicative of a problem in visual filtering and discrimination—i.e., filtering out extraneous stimuli and selecting visual details from a complex field. It is interesting that Witkin et al. (1971), who developed the Embedded Figures Test, felt that poor performance on his test reflects strong field dependency, in which perceptions of individual details are strongly influenced by the surrounding context. Witkin et al. believed that strong field dependency tends to be associated with poor psychological differentiation. This explanation would fit with the identity diffusion and poor sense of interpersonal boundaries commonly described in borderline patients.

Examination of the results of memory testing from all four studies suggests memory problems in both the visual and the auditory/verbal realms. However, given the differing results, it is difficult to assess whether the problem is limited to complex material or may be apparent on both simple and complex retrieval tasks. It is also difficult to determine whether the primary problem lies in initial learning/encoding or in retrieval. Neither the dimension of immediate versus delayed memory nor the dimension of deliberate versus incidental memory appears to explain the memory problem. Nonetheless, these preliminary results suggest that the memory difficulties may not be confined to emotion-laden, conflictual material in borderline patients but rather may represent a broader deficit in memory. Such a memory deficit may contribute to the difficulties borderline patients experience in maintaining a continuous sense of self and in using the past to respond to present events and predict future consequences.

Although we have some better idea of the neuropsychological impairments that borderline patients experience, we know little about the etiology of these impairments. It is possible that many of the manifestations of BPD—including the neuropsychological findings—derive from a fundamental organic impairment. Neuropsychological tests evaluate a number of functions, but very few of the tests are specific to a particular brain site. We see evidence of diffuse brain dysfunction in that both the WAIS-R Digit Symbol (Hirschenfang 1960) and the Embedded Figures (Corkin 1979) are reportedly most sensitive to diffuse dysfunction. In addition, the results do not fit a clear localizing pattern. We found poor performance on tasks linked to both the dominant temporal lobe in the WMS Logical Memory stories (Delaney et al. 1980; Frisk 1988; Milner 1967, 1971) and the nondominant temporal lobe in the Rey-Osterrieth (Taylor 1969) and the Embedded Figures (Corkin 1979). Moreover, it appears that different kinds and sites of organic dysfunction can result in impairments on these tests (Corkin 1979; Kolb and Whishaw 1985; Lezak 1983).

In addition to explanations suggesting constitutionally based organic impairment, it is also possible that subtle neuropsychological impairment may be associated with severe childhood trauma. The estimates of physical and/or sexual abuse in this population range from 40% to 70% (Herman et al. 1989; Ogata et al. 1990; Westen et al. 1990c; Zanarini et al. 1989). It is plausible that severe abuse early in childhood development, with or without a constitutional predisposition, could lead to neuropsychological difficulties in processing information and in memory, through a process of direct brain injury or of emotional kindling (Post and Kopanda 1976; Post et al. 1984). Teicher and colleagues expand on this concept in Chapter 9 of this volume. Although none of the neuropsychological studies described examined abuse history in relation to their findings, abuse may be an important intervening variable.

It is possible that these spotty and diffuse neuropsychological findings are related to the phenomenon of dissociation, separate and apart from the question of abuse. New findings point to a high frequency of dissociation even among those borderline subjects who have not been abused (Zweig-Frank et al. 1993). Since dissociative defenses seem to be very frequent in this disorder, it is possible that they contribute to visuospatial processing problems as well as memory lapses. However, our study, as well as the studies by Carpenter et al. (1993) and Judd and Ruff (1993), contained measures of attention on which borderline subjects showed no differences from healthy control subjects. If dissociation were occurring frequently during testing, it is likely that this would have been reflected on attention measures. Nonetheless, without fuller examination of this question, it cannot be ruled out.

A similar argument can be made against attributing the results to affective dysregulation. It may be that the dysregulation occurs first in this disorder, leading to sensitization to certain stimuli and subsequent erratic responses. If, however, erratic borderline performance were entirely dependent upon labile mood and anxiety states during testing, results might be expected to show a much greater range of responses with wider standard deviations in the borderline group than the reasonably consistent pattern of significant and replicated findings described here.

This is not to say that memory lapses and perceptual distortions are never conflict-driven or defensive in nature. Nonetheless, the findings presented here should lead clinicians who encounter memory lapses and perceptual distortions in their borderline patients to at least consider that these individuals may have a fundamental neuropsychological problem. Certainly, both the psychological and the neuropsychological play a part in many situations for these individuals.

Regardless of etiology, a psychoeducational approach in treatment may be useful. It may prove therapeutic for a clinician to suggest that cognitive processing problems are part of this disorder and that a patient may have "misread" a scene or "forgotten" some important elements of a story. As in all psychoeducational approaches that use a biological or neurological framework to understand a disorder, the goal is not to absolve patients of responsibility for their actions or lapses, but rather to increase patients' awareness of their own predilections so that they can cope with their vulnerabilities and change their behavior.

Therapists may find that encouraging patient use of self-ratings, notes, and journals can facilitate recall in a manner similar to a patient's use of transitional objects to cue evocative memory. If we build upon our findings in which cueing with directed questions regarding forgotten story elements produced a significant number of forgotten details, then perhaps a similar cueing technique may be useful in therapy—for example, "Do you remember, when this happened before, what you did?" Of course, the demarcation between providing cues and "leading the witness" must be kept in mind.

An interesting technique that addressed both memory problems and auditory distortions was used by Orne, the psychiatrist who treated the poet Anne Sexton (Middlebrook 1991). The motivation for those famous psychotherapy tapes was to educate the patient regarding distortions and memory lapses. Following each psychotherapy session, Ms. Sexton would write a full description of the session. The next day, she would return to the therapist's office, without the therapist present, and listen to a tape recording of the actual session. Then she would make notes on the differences between her memories of what had transpired and the actual interaction and discuss the discrepancies in her next session. Ms. Sexton may or may not have been borderline, and the technique may be too labor-intensive for many patients; nonetheless, it is a thorough method of clinically addressing these impairments.

FUTURE RESEARCH DIRECTIONS

Future studies should, we believe, attend to the elements listed in Table 7–2. Ideally, patients should be carefully diagnosed with a standardized instrument and should be medication free. The tests administered should include measures of IQ, attention, and psychomotor skill. It would be extremely useful to study performance in both male and female borderline patients. Drug and alcohol use, along with prior history of attention disorder, should be recorded and taken into consideration when interpreting results. Although the notion that BPD is a subvariant of affective disorder seems to be falling from favor (Gunderson and Phillips 1991), the role of affective symptoms should be considered because of the known effects of depression on neuropsychological functioning.

There is a need for well-chosen comparison groups from the spectrum of other personality disorders and the spectrum of affective disorders. We do not know from the studies reported here whether this pattern of impairment on memory and visuospatial tasks is particular to borderline patients. Findings indicative of diffuse brain injury and of various memory and perceptual deficits may pertain to all personality disorders, or they may be a gross reflection of general psychopathology. On the other hand, these findings may derive not from the disorder of borderline personality, but from other factors that influence the "common pathway" leading to this disorder—for instance, trauma, abuse, and dissociation.

From this preliminary research have emerged questions regarding the relative role of encoding and retrieval in memory impairment. Still unaddressed are questions regarding sequential processing in this patient group. Whether affect-laden material will present more of a memory or a visuospatial problem is another intriguing question. Burgess (1991) has started to examine the relationship between borderline neurocognitive deficits and borderline self-injury. The relationship between these neuropsychological deficits and other symptomatology needs further consideration. The exploration of borderline neuropsychological impairments and the type of object relations impairments being studied by Westen and colleagues (1990a, 1990b; Baker et al. 1992; Stuart et al. 1990) appears to be a rich area for future research. It is to be hoped that past efforts combined with future informed research will provide us with a clearer idea of what occurs within the maze of these patients' cognitive experiences.

REFERENCES

Adler G, Buie DH: Aloneness and borderline psychopathology: the possible relevance of child development issues. Int J Psychoanal 60:83–96, 1979

Amado H, Lustman PJ: Attention deficit disorders persisting in adulthood: a review. Compr Psychiatry 23:300–314, 1982

American Psychiatric Association: Diagnostic and Statistical Manual of Mental Disorders, 3rd Edition. Washington, DC, American Psychiatric Association, 1980

Andrulonis PA, Glueck BC, Stroebel CF, et al: Organic brain dysfunction and the borderline syndrome. Psychiatr Clin North Am 4:47–66, 1981

Andrulonis PA, Glueck BC, Stroebel CF, et al: Borderline personality subcategories. J Nerv Ment Dis 170:670–679, 1982

Armstrong J, Silber JL, Parente FJ: Patterns of thought disorder on psychological testing: implications for adolescent psychopathology. J Nerv Ment Dis 174:448–456, 1986

Baker L, Silk KR, Westen D, et al: Malevolence, splitting, and parental ratings by borderlines. J Nerv Ment Dis 180:258–264, 1992

Berg JL: Differentiating ego functions of borderline and narcissistic personalities. J Pers Assess 55:537–548, 1990

Blatt SJ, Ritzler BA: Thought disorder and boundary disturbance in psychosis. J Consult Clin Psychol 42:370–381, 1974

Burgess JW: Cognitive information processing in borderline personality disorder: a neuropsychiatric hypothesis. Jefferson J Psychiatry 8:34–49, 1990

Burgess JW: Relationship of depression and cognitive impairment to self-injury in borderline personality disorder, major depression, and schizophrenia. Psychiatry Res 38:77–87, 1991

Carpenter CJ, Gold JM, Fenton WS: Neuropsychological testing results in borderline inpatients. Paper presented at the 146th annual meeting of the American Psychiatric Association, San Francisco, CA, May 22–27, 1993

Carr AC, Goldstein EG: Approaches to the diagnosis of borderline conditions by use of psychological tests. J Pers Assess 45:563–574, 1981

Carr AC, Goldstein EG, Hunt HF, et al: Psychological tests and borderline patients. J Pers Assess 43:582–590, 1979

Christman DM: Notes on learning disabilities and the borderline personality. Clinical Social Work Journal 12:18–30, 1984

Cohen DJ, Shaywitz SE, Young JG: Borderline syndromes and attention deficit disorders of childhood: clinical and neurochemical perspectives, in The Borderline Child: Approaches to Etiology, Diagnosis, and Treatment. Edited by Robson KS. New York, McGraw-Hill, 1983, pp 197–221

Corkin S: Hidden-figures-test performance: lasting effects of unilateral penetrating head injury and transient effects of bilateral cingulotomy. Neuropsychologia 17:585–605, 1979

Cornelius JR, Brenner RP, Soloff PH, et al: EEG abnormalities in borderline personality disorder: specific or nonspecific. Biol Psychiatry 21:974–977, 1986

Cornelius JR, Soloff PH, George AWA, et al: An evaluation of the significance of selected neuropsychiatric abnormalities in the etiology of borderline personality disorder. Journal of Personality Disorders 3:19–25, 1989

Cowdry RW, Pickar D, Davies R: Symptoms and EEG findings in the borderline syndrome. Int J Psychiatry Med 15:201–211, 1985–1986

Delaney RC, Rosen AJ, Mattson RH, et al: Memory function in focal epilepsy: a comparison of non-surgical, unilateral temporal lobe, and frontal lobe samples. Cortex 16:103–117, 1980

Edell W: Role of structure and disordered thinking in borderline and schizophrenic disorders. J Pers Assess 51:23–41, 1987

Eich JE: The cue dependent nature of state dependent retrieval. Memory and Cognition 8:157–173, 1980

Eich JE, Weingartner H, Stillman RC, et al: State-dependent accessibility of retrieval cues in the retention of a categorized list. Journal of Verbal Learning and Verbal Behavior 14:408–417, 1975

Exner JE: Some Rorschach data comparing schizophrenics with borderline and schizotypal personality disorders. J Pers Assess 50:455–471, 1986

Fisher S: Some observations suggested by the Rorschach test concerning the ambulatory schizophrenic. Psychiatr Q 29 (suppl):81–89, 1955

Forer BR: The latency of latent schizophrenia. Journal of Projective Techniques 14:297–302, 1950

Frisk V: Comprehension and recall of stories following left temporal lobectomy. Unpublished dissertation, McGill University, Montreal, Canada, 1988

Gabbard GO: Splitting in hospital treatment. Am J Psychiatry 146:444–451, 1989

Gardner DL, Lucas PB, Cowdry RW: Soft sign neurological abnormalities in borderline personality disorder and normal control subjects. J Nerv Ment Dis 175:177–180, 1987

Gittelman R, Mannuzza S, Shenker R, et al: Hyperactive boys almost grown up, I: psychiatric status. Arch Gen Psychiatry 42:937–947, 1985

Grinker RR, Werble B, Drye RC: The Borderline Syndrome: A Behavioral Study of Ego Functions. New York, Basic Books, 1968

Gruenewald D: A psychologist's view of the borderline syndrome. Arch Gen Psychiatry 23:181–184, 1970

Gunderson JG, Phillips KA: A current view of the interface between borderline personality disorder and depression. Am J Psychiatry 148:967–975, 1991

Gunderson JG, Singer MT: Defining borderline patients: an overview. Am J Psychiatry 132:1–10, 1975

Gunderson JG, Kolb JE, Austin V: The diagnostic interview for borderline patients. Am J Psychiatry 138:896–903, 1981

Hartocollis P: The syndrome of minimal brain dysfunction in young adult patients. Bull Menninger Clin 32:102–114, 1968

Heaton RK: A Manual for the Wisconsin Card Sorting Test. Odessa, FL, Psychological Assessment Resources, 1981

Herman JL, Perry JC, van der Kolk BA: Childhood trauma in borderline personality disorder. Am J Psychiatry 146:490–495, 1989

Hirschenfang S: A comparison of WAIS scores of hemiplegic patients with and without aphasia. J Clin Psychol 16:351–352, 1960

Hymowitz P, Hunt HF, Carr AC, et al: The WAIS and Rorschach test in diagnosing borderline personality. J Pers Assess 47:588–596, 1983

Judd PH, Ruff RM: Neuropsychological dysfunction in borderline personality disorder. Journal of Personality Disorders 7:275–284, 1993

Kernberg O: Borderline Conditions and Pathological Narcissism. New York, Jason Aronson, 1975

Kolb B, Whishaw IQ: Fundamentals of Human Neuropsychology. New York, WH Freeman, 1985

Kroll J: The Challenge of the Borderline Patient. New York, WW Norton, 1988

Lerner PM: Rorschach assessment of primitive defenses: a review. J Pers Assess 54:30–46, 1990

Lewinsohn PM, Rosenbaum M: Recall of parental behavior by acute depressives, remitted depressives, and nondepressives. J Pers Soc Psychol 52:611–619, 1987

Lezak MD: Neuropsychological Assessment, 2nd Edition. New York, Oxford University Press, 1983

Lie N: Follow-ups of children with attention deficit hyperactivity disorder. Acta Psychiatr Scand/Suppl 85:1–40, 1992

Lucas PB, Gardner DL, Cowdry RW, et al: Cerebral structure in borderline personality disorder. Psychiatry Res 27:111–115, 1989

Mannuzza S, Klein RG, Konig PH, et al: Hyperactive boys almost grown up, IV: criminality and its relationship to psychiatric status. Arch Gen Psychiatry 46:1073–1079, 1989

Mannuzza S, Klein RG, Bonagura N, et al: Hyperactive boys almost grown up, V: replication of psychiatric status. Arch Gen Psychiatry 48:77–83, 1991

McCully RS: Certain theoretical considerations in relation to borderline schizophrenia and the Rorschach. Journal of Projective Techniques 26:404–418, 1962

Mercer M, Wright SC: Diagnostic testing in a case of latent schizophrenia. Journal of Projective Techniques 14:287–296, 1950

Middlebrook DW: Anne Sexton: A Biography. Boston, MA, Houghton Mifflin, 1991

Milner B: Brain mechanisms suggested by studies of temporal lobes, in Brain Mechanisms Underlying Speech and Language. Edited by Darley FL, Millikan CH. Orlando, FL, Grune & Stratton, 1967

Milner B: Interhemispheric differences in the localization of psychological processes in man. Br Med Bull 27:272–277, 1971

Money J: The Standardized Road-Map Test of Direction Sense: Manual. San Rafael, CA, Acad Therapy, 1976

Muller RJ: Is there a neural basis for borderline splitting? Compr Psychiatry 33:92–104, 1992

Ogata SN, Silk KR, Goodrich S, et al: Childhood sexual and physical abuse in adult patients with borderline personality disorder. Am J Psychiatry 147:1008–1013, 1990

O'Leary KM, Brouwers P, Gardner DL, et al: Neuropsychological testing of patients with borderline personality disorder. Am J Psychiatry 148:106–111, 1991

Osterrieth PA: Le test de copie d'une figure complexe. Archives de Psychologie 30:206–356, 1944

Patrick J, Wolfe B: Rorschach presentation of borderline personality disorder: primary process manifestations. J Clin Psychol 39:442–447, 1983

Post RM, Kopanda RT: Cocaine, kindling, and psychosis. Am J Psychiatry 133:627–634, 1976

Post RM, Rubinow DR, Ballenger JC: Conditioning, sensitization, and kindling: implications for the course of affective illness, in Neurobiology of Mood Disorders. Edited by Post RM, Ballenger JC. Baltimore, MD, Williams & Wilkins, 1984, pp 432–466

Quitkin F, Klein DF: Two behavioral syndromes in young adults related to possible minimal brain dysfunction. J Psychiatr Res 7:131–142, 1969

Rapaport D, Gill MM, Schafer R: Diagnostic Psychological Testing. Edited by Holt R. New York, International Universities Press, 1968 (originally published 1945–1946)

Reitan RM: Trailmaking test results for normal and brain-damaged children. Percept Mot Skills 33:575–581, 1971

Reitan RM, Davison LA: Clinical Neuropsychology: Current Status and Applications. New York, Winston-Wiley, 1974

Rorschach H: Psychodiagnostics, 8th Edition. Translated by Lemkau P, Kronenberg B. New York, Grune & Stratton, 1975 (originally published 1921; revised 1942)

Royer FL: Information processing of visual figures in the digit symbol substitution test. J Exp Psychol 87:335–343, 1971

Ruff RM, Light RH, Evans R: The Ruff figural fluency test: a normative study with adults. Developmental Neuropsychology 3:37–51, 1987

Schafer R: The Clinical Application of Psychological Tests. New York, International Universities Press, 1948

Schafer R: Psychoanalytic Interpretation in Rorschach Testing. New York, Grune & Stratton, 1954

Seashore CE, Lewis D, Saetveit JG: Manual of Instructions and Interpretations for the Seashore Measures of Musical Talents. New York, Psychological Corporation, 1960

Shapiro D: Special problems in testing borderline patients, in A Rorschach Reader. Edited by Sherman MH. New York, International Universities Press, 1960 (originally published 1954)

Singer MT: The borderline diagnosis and psychological tests: review and research, in Borderline Personality Disorders. Edited by Hartocollis P. New York, International Universities Press, 1977, pp 192–213

Singer MT, Larson DG: Borderline personality and the Rorschach test. Arch Gen Psychiatry 38:693–698, 1981

Snyder S, Pitts WM Jr: Electroencephalography of DSM-III borderline personality disorder. Acta Psychiatr Scand 69:129–134, 1984

Snyder S, Pitts WM Jr, Gustin Q: CT scans of patients with borderline personality disorder (letter). Am J Psychiatry 140:272, 1983

Stone MH: The Borderline Syndromes: Constitution, Adaptation and Personality. New York, McGraw-Hill, 1980

Stone HK, Dellis NP: An exploratory investigation into the levels hypothesis. Journal of Projective Techniques 24:333–340, 1960

Street RF: A Gestalt Completion Test: Contributions to Education 481. New York, Columbia University Teachers College, Bureau of Publications, 1931

Strub RL, Black FW: The Mental Status Examination in Neurology. Philadelphia, PA, FA Davis, 1987

Stuart J, Westen D, Lohr N, et al: Object relations in borderlines, depressives, and normals: an examination of human responses on the Rorschach. J Pers Assess 55:296–318, 1990

Taylor LB: Localization of cerebral lesions by psychological testing. Clinical Neurosurgery 16:269–287, 1969

Wechsler D: Wechsler Adult Intelligence Scale—Revised. New York, Psychological Corporation, 1981

Wechsler D: Wechsler Memory Scale—Revised. New York, Psychological Corporation, 1987

Wechsler D, Stone CP: Wechsler Memory Scale Manual. New York, Psychological Corporation, 1945

Weiner IB: Psychodiagnosis in Schizophrenia. New York, Wiley, 1966

Weiss G: Hyperactivity: overview and new directions. Psychiatr Clin North Am 8:737–753, 1985

Wender PH, Reimherr FW, Wood DR: Attention deficit disorder ("minimal brain dysfunction") in adults: a replication study of diagnosis and drug treatment. Arch Gen Psychiatry 38:449–456, 1981

Wender PH, Reimherr FW, Wood DR, et al: A controlled study of methylphenidate in the treatment of attention deficit disorder, residual type, in adults. Am J Psychiatry 142:547–552, 1985

Westen D, Lohr N, Silk KR, et al: Object relations and social cognition in borderlines, major depressives, and normals: a thematic apperception test analysis. Psychological Assessment 2:355–364, 1990a

Westen D, Ludolph P, Silk K, et al: Object relations in borderline adolescents and adults: developmental differences. Adolesc Psychiatry 17:360–384, 1990b

Westen D, Ludolph P, Misle B, et al: Physical and sexual abuse in adolescent girls with borderline personality disorder. Am J Orthopsychiatry 60:55–66, 1990c

Widiger TA: Psychological tests and the borderline diagnosis. J Pers Assess 46:227–238, 1982

Wilson A: Boundary disturbance in borderline and psychotic states. J Pers Assess 49:346–355, 1985

Witkin HA, Oltman PK, Raskin E, et al: A Manual for the Embedded Figures Tests. Palo Alto, CA, Consulting Psychologists Press, 1971

Wood DR, Reimherr FW, Wender P, et al: Diagnosis and treatment of minimal brain dysfunction in adults. Arch Gen Psychiatry 33:1453–1460, 1976

Zanarini MC, Gunderson JG, Marino MF, et al: Childhood experiences of borderline patients. Compr Psychiatry 30:18–25, 1989

Zucker L: The psychology of latent schizophrenia. Am J Psychother 6:44–62, 1952

Zweig-Frank H, Paris JF, Guzder J: Dissociation in female patients with BPD. Paper presented at the 146th annual meeting of the American Psychiatric Association, San Francisco, CA, May 22–27, 1993

Chapter 8

Neurological Dysfunction in Borderline Patients and Axis II Control Subjects

Mary C. Zanarini, Ed.D.
Catherine R. Kimble, M.D.
Amy A. Williams, B.S.

Stern (1938) was the first author to use the term *borderline* to describe a specific pathological condition—a condition that he thought had both neurotic and psychotic features. Since that time, there have been seven main conceptualizations of this term. The first of these conceptualizations is based on the work of Kernberg (1975). In this view, the term borderline is used to describe the most serious forms of character pathology. In the second conceptualization, which reflects the work of Gunderson (1984), borderline refers to a specific form of personality disorder that can be distinguished from a substantial number of other Axis II disorders, particularly those in the "odd" and "anxious" clusters of DSM-III (American Psychiatric Association 1980) and DSM-III-R (American Psychiatric Association 1987). The third conceptualization, which flourished from the 1950s through the early 1970s, focused on the propensity of borderline patients to have transient psychotic or psychotic-like experiences. In this view, borderline personality was considered to be a schizophrenia spectrum disorder (Wender 1977). The fourth conceptualization of the borderline term organized and influenced much of the

---

This study was supported in part by National Institute of Mental Health Grant 1 R29 MH47588-01A1 (Dr. Zanarini).

clinical care and empirical research in the 1980s; it highlighted the chronic dysphoria and affective lability of borderline patients. In this view, borderline personality was thought of as an affective spectrum disorder (Akiskal 1981; Stone 1980).

More recently, it has been proposed that borderline personality disorder (BPD) is best conceptualized as a trauma spectrum disorder because of the high rates of childhood physical and sexual abuse found in borderline subjects in a number of studies (Herman et al. 1989; Links et al. 1988; Ogata et al. 1990; Shearer et al. 1990; Westen et al. 1990; Zanarini et al. 1989a). It has also lately been suggested that BPD is an impulse spectrum disorder—that is, a disorder related to substance use disorders, antisocial personality disorder, and perhaps eating disorders (Zanarini 1993).

More than a decade ago, Andrulonis and his colleagues (Andrulonis and Vogel 1984; Andrulonis et al. 1981, 1982) postulated that at least a subset of borderline patients could best be conceptualized as having some type of organic impairment. Through a chart review, they found that 14% of their nonschizotypal borderline patients had a history of head trauma, encephalitis, or epilepsy, and that 26% had a history of attention-deficit disorder and/or a learning disability (ADD/LD). They also found that patients with BPD were significantly more likely than affective disorder (but not schizophrenic) control subjects to have a history of organic disturbance (both subcategories combined). In addition, they discovered that a significantly higher percentage of male than of female borderline patients had a history of organic disturbance (52% versus 29%) as well as a history of ADD/LD (40% versus 14%). Male borderline patients were also significantly more likely than female borderline patients to engage in antisocial acting out, whereas female borderline patients were significantly more likely than male borderline patients to have a history of depression and eating disorders. Moreover, ADD/LD borderline patients of both sexes engaged in significantly more acting out in an antisocial manner than did nonorganic borderline patients (a finding that was not true for those in either control group).

Surprisingly, this hypothesis has received relatively little empirical investigation. More specifically, only one study has assessed the neurodevelopmental histories of a rigorously defined sample of borderline patients, four studies have examined electroencephalogram (EEG) findings of criteria-defined borderline patients, and three others have investigated structural brain pathology by means of computed tomography (CT) in samples of well-defined borderline patients.

Soloff and Millward (1983) compared the retrospectively obtained neurodevelopmental histories of 45 borderline, 32 depressed, and 42 schizophrenic patients. Although a cumulative tally of neurodevelopmental difficulties failed to demonstrate significant differences between borderline patients and either depressed or schizophrenic control subjects, complications of pregnancy (when pregnant with the "future" borderline) were reported significantly more often by the mothers of borderline patients than by the mothers of depressed or schizophrenic patients. Learning difficulties were reported significantly more often by schizophrenic patients than by borderline patients and significantly more often by borderline patients than by depressed control subjects. However, the generalizability of Soloff and Millward's findings is limited because their study specifically excluded patients with histories of known seizures or other neurological abnormalities.

Electrophysiological dysfunction as measured by EEG findings has been studied in borderline patients because some of the symptoms common in BPD are also common in temporal lobe dysrhythmias—for example, depersonalization, derealization, impulsivity, transient psychosis, and affective lability (Fenwick 1981). Snyder and Pitts (1984) compared the EEG records of 37 male borderline patients with those of 31 male dysthymic control subjects. They found that 19% of the borderline patients had marginally abnormal EEGs and that another 19% had definitely abnormal EEGs. They also found that the rates of definitely abnormal and combined (marginal plus definitely abnormal) EEGs were significantly higher in borderline patients than in dysthymic control subjects. In addition, slow-wave activity was significantly more common in borderline patients than in dysthymic control subjects. Cowdry et al. (1985–1986) studied the EEG records of 39 borderline patients and 20 depressed control subjects and found that definite abnormalities were significantly more common in the EEG records of borderline patients than in those of depressed control subjects (46% versus 10%). They also found that some type of posterior sharp activity was present in a significantly higher percentage of the EEG records of borderline patients than in those of depressed control subjects (41% versus 5%). Cornelius et al. (1986) compared the EEG records of 69 borderline patients and 22 Axis II control subjects and found that there was no statistical difference in the percentage of borderline patients and personality disorder control subjects (19% versus 9%) who had EEG dysrhythmias of all severities. Cornelius et al. (1988) later studied the relationship between clinical symptoms and computerized EEG spectral analysis in 16 borderline patients both before and after amphetamine challenge. They found that mean frequency values on spectral analysis of EEG recordings consistently correlated with anxiety levels but did not correlate with more important symptomatic aspects of BPD.

As discussed by Goyer et al. in Chapter 6 of this volume, the interest in neuroimaging in borderline patients probably arose from the fact that studies of CT scans of the brains of schizophrenic patients have revealed a number of structural abnormalities, including lateral ventricular enlargement as measured by ventricular/brain ratios (VBRs), third ventricular enlargement, and prefrontal atrophy (Raz and Raz 1990). Snyder et al. (1983) found no abnormalities in the CT scans of 26 male borderline patients. Schulz et al. (1983) studied the VBRs of three groups of adolescent patients: 15 schizophrenia/schizophreniform disorder patients, 8 BPD patients, and 18 mixed control subjects. They found that the borderline patients and the mixed control subjects had basically normal VBRs, whereas the schizophrenia spectrum patients had significantly enlarged ventricles. Lucas et al. (1989) studied the CT scans of 31 borderline patients and 28 healthy control subjects on measures of VBR, third ventricle size, and evidence of frontal lobe atrophy. They found that 13% of the patients with BPD and 14% of the control subjects showed some type of structural abnormality. There were no significant differences in any of the measures studied except for a narrower third ventricle in the borderline patients, which the authors speculate may be accounted for by the narrower third ventricle observed in their female patients generally.

To the best of our knowledge, no study has systematically assessed the results of routine neurological examinations of a sample of criteria-defined borderline patients. However, Gardner et al. (1987) administered a "soft sign" neurological examination to 17 borderline patients and 22 nonpsychiatrically ill control subjects (all 39 subjects were women). Neurological soft signs are abnormal motor or sensory findings on neurological examination that are not associated with a specific focal lesion. Their presence suggests—but certainly does not definitely indicate—abnormal neurological development or a disturbance in brain organization or function. Compared with the control subjects, the borderline patients were found to have a significantly greater number of soft sign neurological abnormalities. More specifically, 65% of the borderline patients versus 32% of the control subjects had at least two of the soft signs studied, 47% versus 14% had at least three soft signs, and 47% versus 9% had four or more soft signs.

THE CURRENT STUDY

The purpose of our study was to assess the rate and type of neurological dysfunction in a large sample of criteria-defined borderline patients. This study was designed to build upon earlier studies (i.e., those reviewed above) in four important ways. First, diagnostic assessments were performed with semistructured interviews of demonstrated reliability. Second, control patients meeting DSM-III and/or DSM-III-R criteria for a full range of Axis II disorders were studied. Third, both EEG and CT/magnetic resonance imaging (MRI) reports as well as information concerning neurological examination, seizure history, and head trauma history were obtained. Fourth, information concerning childhood physical and/or sexual abuse—elicited by administering a semistructured interview—was available to determine whether there was any significant relationship between a reported history of childhood abuse and adult neurological dysfunction, a hypothesis most clearly put forward by van der Kolk and Greenberg (1987).

METHOD

This study was part of two larger studies of the phenomenology of BPD. The methodology of the first of these methodologically similar studies has been described elsewhere (Zanarini et al. 1990). Briefly, 296 inpatients at McLean Hospital in Belmont, Massachusetts, participated in these studies. Each patient was initially screened to determine that he or she 1) was between the ages of 18 and 60, 2) had normal or better intelligence, 3) had no history or current symptomatology of a serious organic condition or major psychotic disorder (e.g., schizophrenia or bipolar disorder), 4) had been substance free for at least 10 days, and 5) had been given a definite or probable Axis II diagnosis by the admitting physician or referring clinician. Written informed consent was obtained on all patients. One of us (MCZ), blind to the patients' clinical diagnosis, then evaluated the Axis II status of the first 153 patients by administering the following two research instruments: 1) the Diagnostic Interview for Personality Disorders (DIPD; Zanarini et al. 1987a), a semistructured interview that reliably assesses for the presence of the 11 Axis II disorders described in DSM-III, and 2) the Diagnostic Interview for Borderlines—Revised (DIB-R; Zanarini et al. 1989b), a semistructured interview that can reliably distinguish clinically diagnosed borderline patients from those with other Axis II disorders. The senior author (MCZ) trained two senior psychiatric residents and a clinically experienced research assistant who, also blind to the clinical diagnosis, evaluated the Axis II status of the remaining 134 patients by administering the DIB-R and the Diagnostic Interview for Personality Disorders—Revised (DIPD-R; Zanarini et al. 1987b), the DSM-III-R version of the DIPD.

Information about pathological childhood physical and sexual abuse was obtained by one of three clinically experienced research assistants, each of whom was blind to all other data concerning each patient, including current diagnostic status. This information was assessed with a semistructured interview, the psychometric properties of which have been described elsewhere (Zanarini et al. 1989a). Briefly, this instrument—the Retrospective Family Pathology Questionnaire—inquires about six forms of disturbed behavior chronically engaged in by full-time caregivers. For an item to be given a positive rating, detailed information about the event in question must be provided—for example: "My father used to get drunk just about every weekend and then he would beat my mother and me. This started when I was about 8 or 9 and went on until I left home after high school. He would really punch me and kick me. Sometimes he would pull my hair and try to slam me against a wall."

Information about neurological functioning was assessed through chart review by another author of this chapter (CRK), who was also blind to all diagnostic and childhood information. Neurological examination reports were scored according to the three-point scale of Woods et al. (1986): 2 = focal finding, 1 = nonlocalizing or "soft" finding, and 0 = normal. The neurologist's EEG report was also rated on a three-point scale (2 = focal finding, 1 = nonfocal finding, and 0 = normal finding). The neuroradiologist's CT or MRI reports were grouped together for the purpose of this study, and each report was rated on the following three-point scale: 2 = specific finding, 1 = nonspecific finding, and 0 = normal finding. Seizure histories were obtained by reading the neurology consultant's report, the patient's history as described on the EEG referral form, and the neuropsychology consultant's report. This information was scored on a four-point scale as follows: 3 = clear seizure disorder as evidenced by grand mal seizure history or confirmed spike waves on the EEG, 2 = symptoms or strong suspicion of suspected complex seizure disorder, 1 = withdrawal seizures only, and 0 = normal history (no seizure history). Head injury histories were assessed by reviewing the neurology and/or neuropsychology consultants' reports. This information was scored on the following three-point scale: 2 = severe, with loss of consciousness; 1 = minor, with or without transient loss of consciousness; and 0 = no reported head injuries.

Between-group comparisons involving categorical data were computed with the chi-square statistic corrected for continuity. Independent t tests were used to compute between-group comparisons involving continuous data (age and socioeconomic status). Multivariate analyses were conducted with the forced-entry method of logistic regression.

RESULTS

The charts of all 296 patients were reviewed. Of these patients, 162 met both DIB-R and DSM-III and/or DSM-III-R criteria for BPD, and 134 met DSM-III and/or DSM-III-R criteria for some other type of personality disorder (OPD). Overall, we found that 121, or 74.7%, of the borderline patients and 83, or 61.9%, of the OPD patients had data available on at least one neurological variable. Demographically, these groups were very similar in a number of ways. Both groups had a mean age in the late 20s (28.0 ± 8.0 versus 29.7 ± 8.0) and came, on average, from middle-class backgrounds (mean Hollingshead-Redlich score of 3.1 ± 1.2 versus 2.8 ± 1.2). However, as expected, a significantly higher percentage of borderline patients (76.0%) than Axis II control subjects (43.4%) were women ($\chi^2 = 21.1$, df = 1, $P < .001$).

Table 8–1 shows the number and percentage of borderline and OPD patients with various types of neurological assessments. As can be seen, a significantly higher percentage of borderline patients than of Axis II control subjects had undergone EEGs, CT scans, or MRIs and some type of neurological assessment. However, roughly equal percentages had received a neurological examination, a seizure history, and a head trauma history.

Table 8–2 outlines the number and percentage of each diagnostic group with abnormal findings on each of the measures assessed. As can be seen, these abnormalities were both common

Table 8–1. Percentage of subjects with neurological assessments

Assessment	BPD (N = 162)		OPD (N = 134)	
	n	%	n	%
Neurological examination	105	64.8	78	58.2
EEG	89	54.9	54	40.3[*]
CT/MRI	66	40.7	29	21.6[**]
Seizure history	95	58.6	67	50.0
Head trauma history	87	53.7	59	44.0
Any neurological assessment	121	74.7	83	61.9[*]

Note. BPD = borderline personality disorder. OPD = other personality disorder.
[*]$P < .05$; [**]$P < .001$ (corrected chi-square analyses).

and nondiscriminating, as they were about equally prevalent in borderline patients and Axis II control subjects. Almost 28% of the borderline patients had some type of abnormal finding on routine neurological examination: a focal finding in 7.6% of the patients and a nonlocalizing or "soft" sign in the remaining 20%. Slightly more than 46% of the borderline patients had some type of abnormality on their EEGs: 27.0% had a focal finding and 19.1% had a nonfocal finding. Just over 39% of the borderline patients had some type of abnormality on their CT scans or MRIs:

Table 8–2. Percentage of subjects with positive neurological assessments

Assessment	BPD		OPD	
	n	%	n	%
Neurological examination	29	27.6	15	19.2
Focal finding	8	7.6	1	1.3
Nonfocal finding	21	20.0	14	17.9
EEG	41	46.1	20	37.0
Focal finding	24	27.0	11	20.4
Nonfocal finding	17	19.1	9	16.7
CT/MRI	26	39.4	15	51.7
Specific finding	11	16.7	7	24.1
Nonspecific finding	15	22.7	8	27.6
Seizure history	30	31.6	14	20.9
Clear seizure disorder	11	11.6	1	1.5
Suspected seizure disorder	11	11.6	7	10.4
Withdrawal disorder	8	8.4	6	9.0
Head trauma history	35	40.2	27	45.8
Severe head trauma	17	19.5	14	23.7
Minor head trauma	18	20.7	13	22.0
Any neurological dysfunction	82	67.8	52	62.7

Note. BPD = borderline personality disorder. OPD = other personality disorder.

a specific finding in 16.7% and a nonspecific finding in 22.7%. Almost 32% of the borderline patients had some evidence of a seizure history: 11.6% had a clear seizure disorder as evidenced by a grand mal seizure history or confirmed spike waves on their EEGs, 11.6% had symptoms of or were suspected of having a complex seizure disorder, and 8.4% had had a withdrawal seizure only. Slightly more than 40% of the borderline patients had a history indicative of head trauma: 19.5% had had severe head trauma with loss of consciousness, and 20.7% had had minor head trauma with or without transient loss of consciousness.

Fully 25% of the OPD group met DSM-III and/or DSM-III-R criteria for antisocial personality disorder. All three-way comparisons involving borderline, antisocial, and OPD patients were also nonsignificant.

The relationship between neurological dysfunction and childhood history of abuse was then explored. Of the subjects who had received neurological assessments, 56.2% of the borderline patients and 18.1% of the OPD patients had been physically abused. This difference was strongly statistically significant ($\chi^2 = 29.1$, df = 1, $P < .001$): among this subset, three times as many borderline patients as OPD patients reported a history of physical abuse. Of the subjects who had undergone neurological assessments, 47.9% of the borderline patients and 18.1% of the OPD patients reported a history of sexual abuse. This difference was also highly statistically significant ($\chi^2 = 17.7$, df = 1, $P < .001$), indicating that for this subset, borderline patients were about two to three times as likely as OPD patients to report a childhood history of sexual abuse. However, no comparisons of abused versus nonabused patients with BPD revealed any significant differences in rates of neurological findings or dysfunction. Further, no comparisons of abused borderline patients versus abused OPD patients revealed any significant differences in rates of neurological dysfunction.

Six logistic regressions were also performed, each having age, sex, diagnostic group, childhood history of physical abuse, and childhood history of sexual abuse as the independent variables. The dependent variables were findings (normal/abnormal) on neurological examination, EEG, CT/MRI, seizure history, head trauma history, or any type of neurological assessment. No significant relationships were found in any of these analyses between diagnosis or childhood history of abuse and any of the six types of neurological abnormalities studied.

However, as Table 8–3 shows, borderline patients with a history of physical abuse were significantly more likely than borderline patients who had not reported such a history to have received each of the neurological assessments studied except EEGs. Similarly, borderline patients with a history of sexual abuse were significantly more likely than borderline patients who had not reported such a history to have undergone each of the neurological assessments studied except neurological examinations and EEGs.

DISCUSSION

Three important findings emerge from this study. First, it is quite common for borderline patients to have some form of subtle neurological dysfunction. Second, this dysfunction is not specific to borderline patients, as it is about equally common in near-

Table 8–3. Percentage of abused and nonabused borderline patients with neurological assessments

	Physically				Sexually			
	Abused		Nonabused		Abused		Nonabused	
Assessment	n	%	n	%	n	%	n	%
Neurological examination	59	72.8	46	56.8*	49	71.0	56	60.2
EEG	49	60.5	40	49.4	43	62.3	46	49.5
CT/MRI	41	50.6	25	30.9*	36	52.2	30	32.3*
Seizure history	58	71.6	37	45.7**	50	72.5	45	48.8**
Head trauma history	54	66.7	33	40.7**	46	66.7	41	44.1**
Any neurological assessment	68	84.0	53	65.4**	58	84.1	63	67.7*

Note. Abused versus nonabused BPD patients: *$P < .05$; **$P < .01$ (corrected chi-square analyses).

neighbor Axis II control subjects. Third, neither physical nor sexual abuse in childhood seems to be associated with neurological impairment in adult borderline patients. However, a childhood history of physical and/or sexual abuse seems to be significantly associated with physicians' decisions to order neurological tests on borderline patients.

The results of this study are consistent with previous studies that have shown that neurological dysfunction is common among borderline patients. More specifically, the 46% rate of abnormal EEG findings we found is very similar to the 38% found by Snyder and Pitts (1984) and is identical to the 46% rate of definite abnormal findings found by Cowdry and his colleagues (1985–1986). However, it is substantially higher than the 19% found by Cornelius et al. (1986). This difference may be due to the fact that Cornelius and colleagues excluded patients with seizure histories and recent histories of substance abuse from their sample, whereas these types of patients were included in our more naturalistic study design. Our finding that EEG abnormalities are not specific to borderline patients is consistent with that of Cornelius et al., who also studied Axis II control subjects, but differs from those of Snyder and Pitts and of Cowdry et al., both of whom found that EEG abnormalities were significantly more common among borderline patients than among affective disorder control subjects. This latter finding reinforces the importance of comparing borderline patients with near-neighbor Axis II control subjects, since it is the Axis II patients who share the long-standing patterns of impulsivity, interpersonal difficulties, and circumscribed cognitive disturbances as well as the dysphoria characteristic of borderline patients (Zanarini et al. 1990).

We found that almost 40% of borderline patients who had received a CT scan or an MRI demonstrated some type of structural abnormality. These results stand in contrast to the lack of abnormalities found by Snyder et al. (1983) and Schulz et al. (1983) and to the low rate of 13% found by Lucas et al. (1989). This difference may, in part, be accounted for by the fact that about half of our patients had the more sensitive MRI rather than CT scans. It may also be accounted for by the fact that we were studying a wide range of structural abnormalities, whereas these other investigators were primarily studying ventricular abnormalities found to be common in patients with schizophrenia (Weinberger et al. 1979).

There are almost no studies available with which to compare the other three variables that we explored: neurological examination results, history of seizures, and history of head trauma. We found that only 20% of the borderline patients who had received a routine neurological examination showed soft sign abnormalities. In contrast, Gardner and his associates (1987) found that 47%–65% of the borderline patients they studied had from at least two to at least four soft sign abnormalities. This difference may be due, in part, to the fact that our examinations were not standardized. It may also be partly due to the fact that our examinations did not specifically focus on soft signs of neurological dysfunction.

Fully 40% of our patients with BPD who had been asked whether they ever had experienced head trauma did report a positive history of head trauma; this finding contrasts with the 14% of Andrulonis and Vogel's (1984) patients who reported a history of head trauma, encephalitis, or epilepsy. However, only 19.5% of our borderline patients reported a history of severe head trauma with loss of consciousness. This 19.5% is consistent with the 14% found by Andrulonis and Vogel.

Thirty-two percent of our borderline patients who had had a seizure history taken showed some type of seizure activity, with about 12% having a clear seizure disorder and 12% having symptoms of complex partial seizures (the remaining 8% had had withdrawal seizures only). This figure of 12% with definite evidence of seizure disorder is consistent with the 14% of patients reported by Andrulonis and Vogel (1984) as having a history of head trauma, encephalitis, or epilepsy. The finding that 12% of our borderline subjects were strongly suspected of having partial complex seizures is consistent with the 18% ($N = 40$) of borderline inpatients who reported symptoms of complex partial seizures in the study by Shearer et al. (1990), which also looked at childhood abuse and BPD.

The generalizability of our results needs to be tempered by the limitations of our study. The most important limitation was that our results pertain only to a subset of our sample and not to a consecutive series of patients. Although we believe that a wide variety of factors influenced who was sent for neurological testing, we cannot rule out the possibility that those patients who were thought to have some type of neurological impairment were more likely to be sent for assessment. Second, the various reports that formed the basis of our study were dictated by a number of neurologists and neuropsychologists who were responding to routine clinical referrals and who were neither collecting data nor noting findings in any standardized fashion.

Taken together, the results of our study might seem to indicate that Andrulonis et al.'s (1981, 1982; Andrulonis and Vogel 1984) organic hypothesis has little merit, as was recently concluded by Cornelius and associates (1989) after they reviewed all the data in this area collected at their center. However, we believe that Andrulonis et al.'s original view—that there is a subset of primarily male borderline patients who have ADD/LD and who are prone to antisocial behavior—has yet to be adequately tested. In addition, more refined neurological hypotheses have more recently been suggested and very little empirical work has been done to test their validity. For example, Cowdry and associates (Cowdry et al. 1985–1986; Gardner et al. 1987) have suggested that nonfocal abnormalities in borderline patients may reflect underlying central nervous system dysfunction, which in turn may be associated with the development of BPD. A similar argument has been raised by van der Kolk and Greenberg (1987), who suggest that it may be a childhood of physical and/or sexual abuse that leads to a kindling of the limbic system, which in turn contributes to some of the behaviors and attitudes seen as characteristic or even pathognomonic of borderline patients. Our finding that borderline patients with a history of physical and/or sexual abuse were significantly more likely to have received some sort of neurological assessment lends some support to this hypothesis. Physicians may have ordered these tests because they suspected some sort of subtle organicity in these patients or in order to try to determine whether the dissociative symptoms, irritability, and impulsivity common in these patients could be traced to some neurophysiological disturbance (however subtle) that might respond to informed pharmacotherapy.

Clearly, research focusing on more subtle expressions of either constitutional or acquired neurological dysfunction in criteria-defined borderline patients needs to be undertaken. Such research should include the most sophisticated technologies currently available. It also should include a meticulous neurodevelopmental history as well as a careful assessment of the symptoms of temporal lobe dysfunction, which are very similar to the dissociative experiences common in borderline patients (Mesulam 1981). Currently, we are pursuing these three avenues of investigation in a large-scale, longitudinal study of the course of BPD.

REFERENCES

Akiskal HS: Subaffective disorders: dysthymic, cyclothymic and bipolar II disorders in the "borderline" realm. Psychiatr Clin North Am 4:25–46, 1981

American Psychiatric Association: Diagnostic and Statistical Manual of Mental Disorders, 3rd Edition. Washington, DC, American Psychiatric Association, 1980

American Psychiatric Association: Diagnostic and Statistical Manual of Mental Disorders, 3rd Edition, Revised. Washington, DC, American Psychiatric Association, 1987

Andrulonis PA, Vogel NG: Comparison of borderline personality subcategories to schizophrenic and affective disorders. Br J Psychiatry 144:358–363, 1984

Andrulonis PA, Glueck BC, Stroebel CF, et al: Organic brain dysfunction and the borderline syndrome. Psychiatr Clin North Am 4:47–66, 1981

Andrulonis PA, Glueck BC, Stroebel CF, et al: Borderline personality subcategories. J Nerv Ment Dis 170:670–679, 1982

Cornelius JR, Brenner RP, Soloff PH, et al: EEG abnormalities in borderline personality disorder: specific or nonspecific. Biol Psychiatry 21:974–977, 1986

Cornelius JR, Schulz SC, Brenner RP, et al: Changes in EEG mean frequency associated with anxiety and with amphetamine challenge in BPD. Biol Psychiatry 24:587–594, 1988

Cornelius JR, Soloff PH, George AWA, et al: An evaluation of the significance of selected neuropsychiatric abnormalities in the etiology of borderline personality disorder. Journal of Personality Disorders 3:19–25, 1989

Cowdry RW, Pickar D, Davies R: Symptoms and EEG findings in the borderline syndrome. Int J Psychiatry Med 15:201–211, 1985–1986

Fenwick P: EEG studies, in Epilepsy and Psychiatry. Edited by Reynolds EH, Trimble MR. New York, Churchill Livingstone, 1981, pp 242–263

Gardner DL, Lucas PB, Cowdry RW: Soft sign neurological abnormalities in borderline personality disorder and normal control subjects. J Nerv Ment Dis 175:177–180, 1987

Gunderson JG: Borderline Personality Disorder. Washington, DC, American Psychiatric Press, 1984

Herman JL, Perry JC, van der Kolk BA: Childhood trauma in borderline personality disorder. Am J Psychiatry 146:490–495, 1989

Kernberg O: Borderline Conditions and Pathological Narcissism. New York, Jason Aronson, 1975

Links PS, Steiner M, Offord DR, et al: Characteristics of borderline personality disorder: a Canadian study. Can J Psychiatry 33:336–340, 1988

Lucas PB, Gardner DL, Cowdry RW, et al: Cerebral structure in borderline personality disorder. Psychiatry Res 27:111–115, 1989

Mesulam MM: Dissociative states with abnormal temporal lobe EEG: multiple personality and the illusion of possession. Arch Neurol 38:176–181, 1981

Ogata SN, Silk KR, Goodrich S, et al: Childhood sexual and physical abuse in adult patients with borderline personality disorder. Am J Psychiatry 147:1008–1013, 1990

Raz S, Raz N: Structural brain abnormalities in the major psychoses: a quantitative review of the evidence from computerized imaging. Psychol Bull 108:93–108, 1990

Schulz SC, Koller MM, Kishore PR, et al: Ventricular enlargement in teenage patients with schizophrenia spectrum disorder. Am J Psychiatry 140:1592–1595, 1983

Shearer SL, Peters CP, Quaytman MS, et al: Frequency and correlates of childhood sexual and physical abuse histories in adult female borderline inpatients. Am J Psychiatry 147:214–216, 1990

Snyder S, Pitts WM Jr: Electroencephalography of DSM-III borderline personality disorder. Acta Psychiatr Scand 69:129–134, 1984

Snyder S, Pitts WM Jr, Gustin Q: CT scans of patients with borderline personality disorder (letter). Am J Psychiatry 140:272, 1983

Soloff PH, Millward JW: Developmental histories of borderline patients. Compr Psychiatry 24:574–588, 1983

Stern A: Psychoanalytic investigation of and therapy in the borderline group of neuroses. Psychoanal Q 7:467–489, 1938

Stone MH: The Borderline Syndromes: Constitution, Personality, and Adaptation. New York, McGraw-Hill, 1980 van der Kolk BA, Greenberg MS: The psychobiology of the trauma response: hyperarousal, constriction, and addiction to traumatic reexposure, in Psychological Trauma. Edited by van der Kolk BA. Washington, DC, American Psychiatric Press, 1987, pp 63–87

Weinberger DR, Torrey EF, Neophytides AN, et al: Lateral cerebral ventricular enlargement in chronic schizophrenia. Arch Gen Psychiatry 36:735–739, 1979

Wender PH: The contribution of the adoption studies to an understanding of the phenomenology and etiology of borderline schizophrenia, in Borderline Personality Disorders: The Concept, the Syndrome, the Patient. Edited by Hartocollis P. New York, International Universities Press, 1977, pp 255–269

Westen D, Ludolph P, Misle B, et al: Physical and sexual abuse in adolescent girls with borderline personality disorder. Am J Orthopsychiatry 60:55–66, 1990

Woods BT, Kinney DK, Yurgelun-Todd D: Neurologic abnormalities in schizophrenic patients and their families, I: comparison of schizophrenic, bipolar, and substance abuse patients and normal controls. Arch Gen Psychiatry 43:657–663, 1986

Zanarini MC: BPD as an impulse spectrum disorder, in Borderline Personality Disorder: Etiology and Treatment. Edited by Paris J. Washington, DC, American Psychiatric Press, 1993, pp 67–85

Zanarini MC, Frankenburg FR, Chauncey DL, et al: The diagnostic interview for personality disorders: interrater and test–retest reliability. Compr Psychiatry 28:467–480, 1987a

Zanarini MC, Frankenburg FR, Chauncey DL: The revised diagnostic interview for personality disorders. Belmont, MA, McLean Hospital, Psychosocial Research Program, 1987b

Zanarini MC, Gunderson JG, Marino MF, et al: Childhood experiences of borderline patients. Compr Psychiatry 30:18–25, 1989a

Zanarini MC, Gunderson JG, Frankenburg FR, et al: The revised diagnostic interview for borderlines: discriminating BPD from other Axis II disorders. Journal of Personality Disorders 3:10–18, 1989b

Zanarini MC, Gunderson JG, Frankenburg FR, et al: Discriminating borderline personality disorder from other Axis II disorders. Am J Psychiatry 147:161–167, 1990

Chapter 9

Early Abuse, Limbic System Dysfunction, and Borderline Personality Disorder

Martin H. Teicher, M.D., Ph.D.
Yutaka Ito, M.D.
Carol A. Glod, R.N., M.S., C.S.
Fred Schiffer, M.D.
Harris A. Gelbard, M.D., Ph.D.

Borderline personality disorder (BPD) is a serious psychiatric disturbance generally characterized by intense, unstable interpersonal relationships, affective instability, aggression, frequent suicidal thoughts or attempts, and self-destructive behavior. Although BPD is often considered to be the result of abnormal personality development, there is increasing recognition that these symptoms may be suggestive of a state of serotonin dysregulation (Coccaro et al. 1989) or limbic system irritability (Andrulonis et al. 1981). Our aim in this chapter is to provide an integrative biopsychosocial model of BPD that emphasizes the possible deleterious effects of intense adverse early experience on brain development.

PSYCHOLOGICAL EFFECTS OF EARLY ABUSE

Physical and sexual traumatization in childhood is often associated with the development of psychiatric difficulties. The initial sequelae of abuse may manifest as a constellation of internalizing symptoms such as depression, anxiety, suicidal ideation, and posttraumatic stress (Famularo et al. 1988; Finkelhor 1986; Kashani and Carlson 1987) or as an externalizing cluster that includes aggressive impulsivity, delinquency, and substance abuse (A. W. Burgess et al. 1987; Finkelhor 1986). Early abuse is also associated with general psychopathology and increased symptomatology in adults (Bryer et al. 1987). Childhood trauma has been implicated as a factor in the development of somatoform disorder (Krystal 1978) and panic disorder with agoraphobia (Faravelli et al. 1985). Key studies by Stone (1981), Herman and colleagues (Herman 1986; Herman et al. 1989), and others (Links et al. 1988; Ogata et al. 1990; Shearer et al. 1990; Westen et al. 1990; Zanarini et al. 1989) have revealed a strong association between early abuse and the development of BPD. In some studies as many as 81% of patients with definite BPD reported a history of major childhood trauma. Physical abuse occurred in 71% of the borderline subjects, sexual abuse in 67%, and 62% had witnessed domestic violence (Herman et al. 1989). Compared with histories reported by other personality disorder patients, histories of early childhood trauma (0–6 years) were found almost exclusively in borderline patients (Herman et al. 1989). Beck and van der Kolk (1987) have suggested a possible relationship between early sexual abuse and severe, intractable psychotic disorders. Forty-six percent of their sample of chronically institutionalized and actively psychotic female patients reported a history of childhood incest. In addition, many studies have identified a strong link between early abuse and the development of multiple personality disorder (MPD) (Bliss 1980; Horevitz and Braun 1984; Putnam et al. 1986). In a study of 100 MPD patients, Putnam and colleagues (1986) found a history of significant and severe childhood trauma (generally child abuse) in 83% of these patients.

Thus, persistent childhood abuse may be associated with a spectrum of psychiatric disorders in adults. These adult disorders range from the extreme adaptive reactions seen in MPD and refractory psychosis, to intermediate adaptive reactions present in BPD, to more delimited reactions manifest in somatoform and panic disorders (Herman et al. 1989). As we suggest below, this spectrum of psychopathology may stem from different types and degrees of limbic system or cortical dysfunction.

NEURAL REGULATION OF HUMAN EMOTION AND PERSONALITY

Limbic System

The limbic system is a somewhat ill-defined collection of neuroanatomical regions linked via common phylogeny, cytoarchitecture, membrane proteins, and neural connections (Levitt 1984; Lopes da Silva et al. 1990; Reep 1984). In its broadest sense this region consists of the subcallosal, cingulate, and parahippocampal gyri and the underlying hippocampal formation, dentate gyrus, and amygdaloid complex in the temporal lobe; portions of the frontal cortex; the septal nuclei; the hypothalamus; the anterior thalamic nuclei; the olfactory bulbs and tracts; and parts of the basal ganglia (limbic striatum). These components influence memory, learning, emotional states and responses, and behavior, particularly aggressive, oral, and sexual activity and behavior (Pincus and Tucker 1978).

Hippocampus

The hippocampal formation and parahippocampal gyrus have been strongly implicated in the pathophysiology of generalized anxiety and panic disorders (Gray et al. 1983; Reiman et al. 1984; Teicher 1988). These anxiety disorders possibly arise from excess noradrenergic influences on the hippocampus ascending from the locus coeruleus (Gorman et al. 1989). This region also plays a major role in memory (Pincus and Tucker 1978) and is probably a critical locus for the generation of dissociative states (Mesulam 1981). Recent research also suggests that the septal area and the hippocampus are crucial components of the behavioral inhibitory system, which acts to arrest ongoing behavior when it is environmentally inappropriate (Depue and Spoont 1986). The threshold setting—that is, the degree of inhibition versus disinhibition—for this system is modulated by serotonergic projections from the median raphe nuclei (Depue and Spoont 1986). Thus, the hippocampal area may subserve many of the anxiogenic, dissociative, amnestic, and disinhibitory aspects and symptoms associated with posttraumatic stress disorder.

Amygdala

The interconnecting amygdaloid nuclei have been strongly implicated in the control of aggressive, oral, and sexual behaviors (Pincus and Tucker 1978). Irritable foci in the amygdaloid nuclei have been associated with episodic dyscontrol and impulsive violence in humans (Pincus and Tucker 1978). This region is one of the most sensitive structures in the brain for the emergence of kindling, an important phenomenon in which repeated, intermittent stimulation produces greater and greater alteration in neuronal excitability that may eventually result in seizures (Goddard et al. 1969; Post et al. 1984). However, the emergence of seizure activity is not critical to the concept of kindling. Kindling results in long-term alterations in neuronal excitability that can have major impacts on behavioral control (Post et al. 1984). Van der Kolk and Greenberg (1987) have proposed that repeated traumatization—particularly child abuse—may lead to limbic kindling and to the emergence of neurological abnormalities, which can then lead to inappropriate aggression and sexual activity.

Limbic Striatum and Prefrontal Cortex

Important research by Nauta and Domesick (Domesick 1988) have expanded the concept of the limbic system to include the limbic striatum, which receives overlapping limbic projections from the hippocampal formation, the basolateral nucleus of the amygdala, the cingulate cortex, the prefrontal cortex, and the dorsal raphe nuclei. The limbic striatum is densely innervated by dopamine projections from the ventral tegmental area. Enkephalin projections are also found here, and these pathways may have a strong relationship to the addictive components of trauma (van der Kolk and Greenberg 1987). The limbic striatum and associated connections provide a major gateway through which behavioral action can be inhibited or disinhibited (Depue and Spoont 1986). In adults the prefrontal cortex plays a decisive role in controlling activity within this circuit. Damage to the prefrontal cortex, particularly irritative lesions, can produce marked changes in personality with emergence of impulsive behavior, "emotional incontinence," poor self-control, and dulled awareness of the consequences of one's actions (Pincus and Tucker 1978).

The Right Hemisphere and Perception and Expression of Emotion

Several lines of research suggest that the right hemisphere plays a particularly significant role in the perception and expression of emotion. Some authors have theorized that the right hemisphere is specialized for emotional processing in a fashion analogous to the left hemisphere's specialization for language (e.g., Ross 1981). Three basic hypotheses have been advanced. The right hemisphere hypothesis postulates that the right hemisphere is specialized for the perception and expression of essentially all emotions (Borod 1992). The valence hypothesis maintains that the right hemisphere is specialized for the perception and expression of negative emotions, whereas the left hemisphere is specialized for the perception and expression of positive emotions (Silberman and Weingartner 1986; Tomarken et al. 1992). There is also a mixed hemispheric valence hypothesis that proposes that the right hemisphere is dominant for the perception of all emotions and for the expression of negative emotions, while the left hemisphere plays a leading role in the expression of positive emotions (Borod 1992; Hirschman and Safer 1982). Davidson et al. (1990) have suggested that the determining factor is not the positive or negative valence of the emotion, but whether the emotional response is associated with approach or withdrawal. This distinction may be important because certain emotions such as anger can be associated with either approach or withdrawal behaviors (Davidson et al. 1990). Borod (1992) provides an excellent review of studies in this area, which strongly suggest that the right hemisphere plays a dominant role in our capacity to recognize emotion through nonlinguistic visual and auditory channels. Most studies also demonstrate right hemisphere dominance in the expression of both positive and negative emotions, although in this area the data are less compelling (Borod 1992). Under normal circumstances, our capacity to appropriately identify and evaluate the affects of others, and in turn to appropriately communicate our own affects, depends on a healthy interaction between right hemisphere emotional perception and left hemisphere linguistic processing and reason.

Summary of Neural Regulation of Emotion and Personality

It is likely that the anxiogenic, amnestic, somatic, and dissociative effects of trauma are mediated via hippocampal projections in the limbic system and controlled by the neurotransmitter norepinephrine. The inappropriate release of aggressive and sexual behaviors may relate to development of irritative kindled foci in the amygdala or the prefrontal cortex or to deficiencies in serotonin regulation of the septo-hippocampal behavioral inhibitory system. Damage to the right hemisphere can produce a myriad of affective abnormalities, including indifference, depression, hysteria, gross social-emotional disinhibition, florid manic excitement, childishness, euphoria, impulsivity, and abnormal sexual behavior (Joseph 1988). Studies of normal and "split-brain" function suggest that the right hemisphere maintains a highly developed social-emotional mental system and can independently perceive, recall, and act on certain memories and experiences without the aid or active reflective participation of the left hemisphere (Joseph 1988). Lack of or poorly regulated integration of left and right hemisphere function may result in the misperception of affect, and this interhemispheric integration difficulty can foster a situation in which the right and left halves of the brain act in an uncooperative fashion, giving rise to intrapsychic conflict and splitting (Joseph 1988; Muller 1992).

DEVELOPMENTAL CONSIDERATIONS

The prefrontal cortex, hippocampus, and amygdala are among the most of plastic brain regions. The prefrontal cortex has the most delayed ontogeny of any brain region: major projections to the prefrontal cortex scarcely begin to myelinate until adolescence (Alexander and Goldman 1978; Fuster 1980; Goldman 1971; Weinberger 1987). Dopamine projections to the prefrontal cortex are specifically and selectively activated by stress (Deutch et al. 1985; Knorr et al. 1989; Reinhard et al. 1982). Thus, it is conceivable that stress activates the prefrontal cortex and alters its development. We theorize that stress may produce a precocious development of the prefrontal cortex that leads to signs of early maturation (e.g., the "parentified child"), but stress may also arrest the development of this region and prevent it from reaching full adult capacity. The hippocampus is a region in which neurogenesis continues into postnatal life, and the cellular organization of the hippocampus can be markedly affected by levels of corticosteroids, which can produce cell death (Sapolsky et al. 1990). The amygdala is a major site of which overstimulation at any age can result in persistent kindled changes in neuronal excitability and behavior (Post et al. 1984). Cynader et al. (1981) have shown in kittens that the normal bidirectional flow of cortical information through the corpus callosum can be affected by early experience, and in extreme circumstances a situation can result in which communication in the corpus callosum becomes entirely unidirectional. Human research suggests that lateralized differences in frontal cortical activity may be established very early in life and probably play a dominant role in temperamental reactions (Fox and Davidson 1986). Evidence indicates that the degree and direction of lateralized function is determined by genetic, hormonal, and experiential factors (Denenberg 1983; Galin 1977; Joseph 1988; Muller 1992). All of these regions of the brain are probably markedly affected by early abuse and trauma, which sometimes results in persistent neuropsychiatric disturbances manifested by long-term, serious effects on mood, cognition, and behavior.

Effects of Early Abuse on Human Brain Development and Function

Although researchers have long suggested that early deprivation and abuse may result in neurobiological abnormalities (Hofer 1975; Hubel 1978; Teicher 1989), there is very little empirical evidence available to indicate whether this is true in humans (van der Kolk and Greenberg 1987). Many abused children show evidence of neurological damage, even in the absence of apparent or reported head injury. Green et al. (1981) found that soft neurological signs and nonspecific electroencephalogram (EEG) abnormalities were more common in abused children and considered this condition to be an additional source of trauma. The "soft" neurological deficits can amplify the pathological impact of an abusive environment (Green 1983). This subject is discussed in somewhat more detail with respect to borderline patients in Chapter 8 by Zanarini and her colleagues. However, another consequence of abnormal EEG activity (particularly temporal spikes and sharp waves) may be a tendency toward aggressive behavior. Although the relationship between sharp waves and temporal spikes and aggression is controversial, some studies suggest that EEG abnormalities are frequently present in patients who exhibit episodic violence. For instance, in a study of 130 violent patients with substantial histories of childhood deprivation, parental psychiatric illness, and family violence, Bach-y-Rita et al. (1971) found that one-half of all patients who received EEGs showed abnormalities, particularly temporal spikes. EEG abnormalities have also been reported to be a significant risk factor for suicidal ideation or attempts. One of the earliest pioneering studies on the physiological determinants of suicide reported a strong positive association between paroxysmal EEG disturbances and suicidal ideation, suicide attempts, and assaultive-destructive behavior (Struve et al. 1972).

Childhood incest has been associated with reports of abnormal EEG activity. Davies (1978–1979) reported that 77% of 22 patients who had been the child or the younger member of an incestuous relationship had abnormal EEGs, and that 36% of these patients had had clinical seizures. The patients in this study also suffered from impulsivity and depersonalization. Davies (1978–1979) suggested that these children were more at risk for being sexually abused by family members. We suggest, on the other hand, that the trauma of the abuse itself and the need to repress memories of the abuse and to dissociate the affects and perhaps the experience of the abuse may have overwhelmed the developing limbic system and produced these abnormalities.

The relationship among abnormal EEG activity, temporal lobe epilepsy (TLE), dissociative phenomena, and the emergence of MPD is complex and unresolved. Both Mesulam (1981) and

Schenk and Baer (1981) have suggested that there is a strong association among TLE, dissociation, and MPD. However, Coons et al. (1988) reported that significant neurological and EEG abnormalities were "infrequently observed" in patients with MPD. Nonetheless, 23% of their population had grossly abnormal EEGs with paroxysmal spikes and sharp waves; this percentage is about 10 times the reported incidence of paroxysmal EEG events observed in other studies of psychiatric patients (Goodin and Aminoff 1984). Unfortunately, the EEG is an unreliable method for detecting TLE in the interictal period. Even in patients with EEG-verified TLE, only 44% would be expected to have detectable paroxysmal EEG spikes and sharp waves in the interictal period (Goodin and Aminoff 1984; Matthews 1964). Given the low detection rate of TLE by the EEG, Coons et al.'s (1988) study actually shows a remarkably strong association between MPD and TLE. Although some studies suggest that patients with MPD may have limbic system or temporal lobe dysfunction, it is clear that the majority of patients with TLE do not show evidence for MPD or dissociative disorders (Ross et al. 1989). Thus, a temporal lobe seizure focus is not a sufficient cause for the development of MPD. Nevertheless, based on Davies's (1978–1979) report and our own observations (see below), we theorize that patients who were abused in childhood may develop transient temporal lobe electrical abnormalities, and that these neuropsychological disturbances in the context of the abusive experience may serve as a catalyst for the emergence of dissociation and the genesis of multiple personalities or fragments. Thus, childhood abuse may result in EEG abnormalities that persist in some patients into adulthood, but the persistence of EEG abnormalities would not be a necessary consequence. However, alterations in EEG activity have been associated with the emergence of different personalities in MPD (Brende 1984).

Neurological Dysfunction in Patients With Borderline Personality Disorder

Previous research has suggested a possible relationship between BPD and temporal lobe–limbic system dysfunction (Andrulonis et al. 1981; Cowdry et al. 1985–1986; Snyder and Pitts 1984). EEG abnormalities have been studied by Snyder and Pitts (1984), who reported that patients with BPD had a higher incidence of EEG abnormalities (38% abnormal) than a contrast group of dysthymic patients (13% abnormal). Similarly, Cowdry et al. (1985–1986) found that 41% of BPD patients had definite sharp wave abnormalities on EEG, compared with only 5% of patients with unipolar depression ($P < .005$). On the other hand, Cornelius et al. (1986) reported that the incidence of EEG abnormalities in patients with BPD (18.8%) was not statistically significantly higher than that in a control group consisting of patients with other personality disorders (9.1%). In part, this study lacked sufficient statistical power to detect a 100% difference in risk, and more than half of the patients in the control group had mixed personality disorders (which may or may not have had borderline features) and antisocial personality disorder (which shares important clinical features with BPD). Both Cornelius et al. (1986, 1988) and Snyder and Pitts (1984) found no correlation between severity of borderline symptoms and severity of EEG abnormalities. However, looking for such a correlation may be asking much more from conventional, or spectral, EEG than is appropriate.

Recent studies have also found associations between BPD and abnormalities on neuropsychological testing. This topic is reviewed in much more detail by O'Leary and Cowdry in Chapter 7. J. W. Burgess (1992) found that patients with personality disorders in the dramatic cluster (histrionic, narcissistic, borderline, and antisocial) showed evidence of significant deficiencies in neurocognitive performance, particularly in subtests requiring multistep, multi-element associative operations. Similarly, O'Leary et al. (1991) found that patients with BPD were impaired in their ability to extract essential versus extraneous visual information as well as in their capacity to recall complex material. In short, there is reason to suspect that patients with BPD have alterations in corticolimbic function, although it is unlikely, given the relative coarseness of these measures, that those alterations indicate abnormalities specific to BPD. Nevertheless, these findings lend credence to the search for neurobiological abnormalities associated with early abuse that may be related to the emergence of BPD.

NEW RESEARCH

Association Between Early Abuse and Ratings of Limbic Dysfunction in Adulthood

To study the possible relationship between early abuse and limbic system dysfunction, we devised a self-report questionnaire—the Limbic System Checklist—33 (LSCL-33)—to evaluate the frequency with which patients experienced 33 symptom categories often encountered as ictal TLE phenomena (Teicher et al. 1993). The items were taken from the work of Spiers et al. (1985). Broadly, the items on the LSCL-33 checklist can be divided into paroxysmal somatic disturbances, brief hallucinatory events, visual disturbances, automatisms, and dissociative experiences. Subjects rated the lifetime frequency with which they experienced these disturbances according to the predefined descriptors of "never," "rarely," "sometimes," and "often." From these descriptors, a total score was derived. Factor scores for somatic, sensory, behavioral, and mnemonic disturbances were determined as well.

Previous research had shown that LSCL-33 scores were low in nonpsychiatrically ill control subjects (< 10) and elevated in patients with documented TLE (range 23–60). LSCL-33 scores correlated well with scores on the Dissociative Experience Scale (DES; Bernstein and Putnam 1986) ($r = .81$, $n = 16$). LSCL-33 scores also correlated moderately well with the somatization ($r = .65$) and psychoticism ($r = .57$) subscales of the Hopkins Symptom Checklist—90 (SCL-90; Derogatis et al. 1974), although none of the other SCL-90 subscales added to the overall correlation. An intertest interval of 7–14 days was used to evaluate test–retest measures of reliability in 16 individuals with widely different psychiatric diagnoses and backgrounds. The correlation between the two test sessions was high ($r = .92$). Each of the four subscales of the instrument also correlated closely on retesting (somatic $r = .83$, sensory $r = .83$, behavioral $r = .86$, and mnemonic $r = .78$). These preliminary psychometric investigations suggest that the LSCL-33 may be a meaningful survey instrument.

To test for a possible association between early abuse and limbic system dysfunction, we evaluated 253 adult outpatients who presented for assessment at the Adult Outpatient Clinic of McLean Hospital (Belmont, Massachusetts). The mean age of the sample was 34 years (range 17–69), and 58% were female. In addition to the LSCL-33, the Life Experience Questionnaire (LEQ; Bryer et al. 1987) was used to elicit abuse history. Each subject reported the type of abuse experienced (physical and/or sexual), age at onset, duration, and perpetrator of the abuse. Fifty-six percent of patients reported a history of some abuse during their lifetime. Sixteen percent acknowledged both physical and sexual abuse, 30% reported a history of physical abuse only, and 10% reported a history of sexual abuse only.

Overall abuse had a prominent effect on total LSCL-33 scores ($P < .0001$; Figure 9–1). Subjects who indicated that they had never been abused ($n = 109$) had mean LSCL-33 scores of 13.6 ± 11.3. Compared with scores for never-abused subjects, total LSCL-33 scores were 38% higher for patients who had been abused physically but not sexually ($P < .01$, $n = 77$) and 49% higher for patients who had been abused sexually but not physically ($P < .02$, $n = 26$). Patients who acknowledged both physical and sexual abuse ($n = 41$) had scores that were 113% higher than those of patients who did not report abuse ($P < .0001$). LSCL-33 scores from men and women were similarly affected by abuse, although nonabused men had insignificantly lower LSCL-33 scores than did nonabused women.

As expected, abuse before the age of 18 had a greater impact than abuse after age 18. Patients who were sexually but not physically abused before the age of 18 ($n = 20$) had scores that were 66% higher than those of patients who had never been abused ($P < .003$). In contrast, patients who were sexually but not physically abused after age 18 ($n = 6$) had scores that were no different from those of nonabused patients. Similarly, patients who were physically but not sexually abused before age 18 ($n = 45$) had scores that were 52% higher than those of nonabused patients ($P < .004$), whereas patients physically but not sexually abused after age 18 ($n = 29$) had scores that were not significantly higher than nonabused patients. Although age at the time of first abuse was a significant factor for those patients subjected to either physical or sexual abuse, patients who were abused both physically and sexually were strongly affected, regardless of

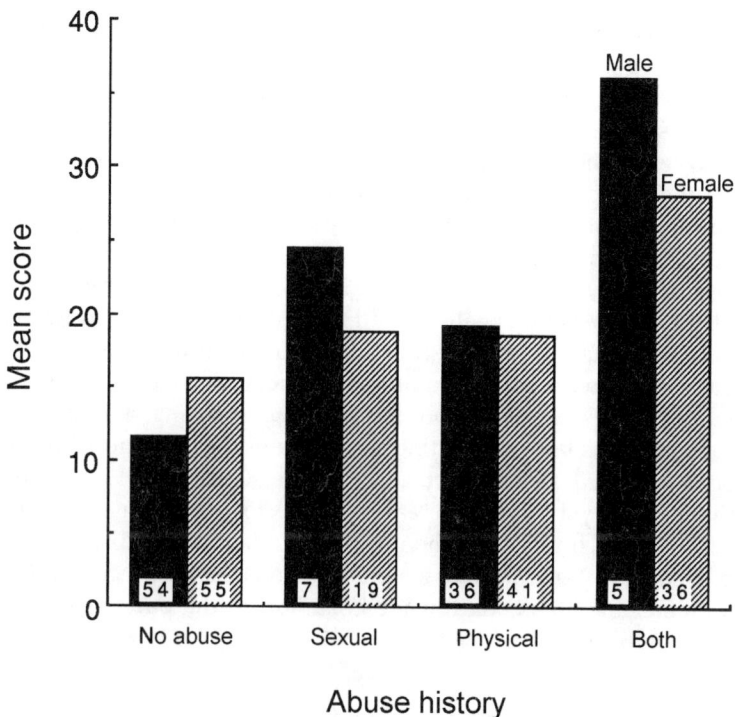

Figure 9–1. Total Limbic System Checklist–33 (LSCL-33; Teicher et al. 1993) scores in adult psychiatric outpatients in relationship to their reported histories of physical or sexual abuse and gender.
Note. Numbers in bars indicate sample size of each group.

their age at first abuse. Hence, patients with combined abuse prior to age 18 ($n = 11$) had scores that were 147% higher than those of nonabused patients ($P < .0001$), whereas patients abused both physically and sexually for the first time after age 18 ($n = 8$) had scores that were 127% higher ($P < .0002$).

Each of the subscale scores of the LSCL-33 was affected by abuse in a similar manner. Each subscale was most markedly elevated in patients with a history of combined physical and sexual abuse, whereas a history of either physical or sexual abuse alone was associated with intermediate scores. Gender differences were present only on the somatic subscale, with women having overall somatic scores 39% greater than those of men ($P <$ .01). There were no significant gender–by–abuse category interactions.

Overall, these findings are consistent with our hypothesis that early childhood abuse is associated with an increased incidence of limbic system dysfunction. However, despite the high association between abuse and LSCL-33 scores, a number of limitations exist in this study. First, the LSCL-33 is a new instrument, and further analysis of its validity and reliability is needed. Confirmation of limbic system dysfunction through more direct assessment of brain function or anatomy is crucial. Second, this study is purely correlational: although it identifies a strong statistical association, no claims regarding a cause-and-effect relationship can be established. It may be true, as Davies (1978–1979) proposed, that limbic dysfunction increases the risk for early abuse. It is also possible that limbic dysfunction may be a hereditary disturbance, passed from generation to generation, and thus is associated with a greater likelihood of abusive behavior on the part of parents, siblings, or relatives.

Association Between Early Abuse and EEG Abnormalities in Childhood

The aim of our second study was to ascertain whether childhood physical, sexual, or psychological abuse was associated with direct evidence of neurobiological abnormalities. A chart review was conducted to blindly examine the association between different categories of abuse and evidence for abnormalities on EEG, brain electrical activity mapping (BEAM), computed tomography (CT), magnetic resonance imaging (MRI), neurological examination, and neuropsychological testing (Ito et al. 1993). We hypothesized that if early abuse affects neurobiological development, an increased rate of abnormalities on some of these tests should be evident. Furthermore, if abuse has relatively specific deleterious neurobiological effects, it may be possible to detect a circumscribed constellation of abnormalities that are significantly more prevalent in abused children.

Medical records were reviewed on 115 consecutive admissions

to a child and adolescent psychiatric hospital that occurred between June 1988 and May 1989. Eleven cases were eliminated because of possible preexisting neurological abnormalities unrelated to abuse. The mean age of the remaining 104 patients was 13.0 years. Sixty percent were adolescents (13 years or older) and 51% were male. Most of the subjects were Caucasian (86%). IQ test scores were above 85 in 84%, and 7% were mildly or moderately retarded (IQ below 71).

The medical records were transcribed by research assistants, who prepared separate sheets for abuse history and neurological results on each subject. These sheets were separated and coded for independent blind scoring by two experienced clinicians. Any discrepant item was reviewed by a third blind clinician. Final scores required identical assessment by two of three raters. Neurological evaluations and tests were ordered based on clinical need, and the specialists who conducted these tests were unaware of our research interests or hypotheses.

Four broad categories of childhood trauma were evaluated: physical abuse, sexual abuse, psychological abuse (witnessing domestic violence, verbal abuse), and neglect. Each category was rated on a three-point scale: 0 = no known abuse or neglect; 1 = possible history of serious abuse or neglect, or known incidence of abuse of moderate severity; and 2 = documented history of serious abuse or neglect. Neurological assessments were divided into four categories: imaging studies (CT or MRI scans), electrophysiological studies (EEG or BEAM), neurological examination, and neuropsychological testing. Results for each category were rated as either normal or abnormal.

Neurological examinations were performed on 96% of the subjects. Ninety percent received electrophysiological assessment, 86% underwent neuropsychological testing, and 67% had neuroimaging studies. Overall, 98% of the neurological assessment categories and 80% of the abuse categories were scored identically by the two assigned clinician raters. All discrepancies were satisfactorily resolved by the blind third rater, who agreed with one of the two discrepant scores.

Subjects were divided into four groups based on abuse scores. Patients in the nonabused group had no evidence of abuse in any of the four categories. Patients in the psychological abuse group had scores of 1 or 2 for psychological abuse or neglect but scores of 0 for physical and sexual abuse. Patients in the overall physical/sexual abuse group had either physical or sexual abuse scores of 1 or 2, regardless of scores for the other categories. Patients in the severe physical/sexual abuse group had physical or sexual abuse scores of 2, indicating a documented history of severe abuse. Based on abuse scores, 27 patients were assigned to the nonabused group, 22 patients to the psychological abuse group, and 55 patients to the overall physical/sexual abuse group. Thirty-eight patients in the physical/sexual abuse group had sustained unequivocal abuse of substantial severity.

Differences among the groups on neurological assessment measures are summarized in Table 9–1. There were no differences between abused and nonabused patients in the prevalence of abnormal neurological exam findings or abnormal neuropsychological test results. Abnormal imaging results were found in 15% of the nonabused patients and in 26% of the abused patients; however, this difference was not statistically significant. Abnormal electrophysiological findings were observed in 26.9% of the nonabused patients but in 54.4% of the patients with a history of early trauma ($P = .021$). Abnormal electrophysiological results were found in 42.9% of the patients with psychological abuse, in 59.6% of the total sample with physical/sexual abuse ($P = .014$), and in 71.9% of the subsample with serious physical/sexual abuse ($P = .0013$). As seen in Table 9–2, the overall prevalence of abnormal electrophysiological results in patients with a significant history of abuse or neglect was about the same (53.3%–56.3%) regardless of age or gender. The psychological abuse group and the physical/sexual abuse group had statistically comparable prevalences of abnormal electrophysiological results (42.9% versus 59.6%) (Table 9–1).

The majority of abnormal electrophysiological results occurred in frontotemporal or anterior regions (Table 9–3). In the nonabused group, 19.2% of the patients had abnormalities within this area, whereas 47% of the abused patients had electrophysiological abnormalities in this region ($P = .018$). Patients with a history of physical/sexual abuse had a 3- to 4-fold greater prevalence of EEG abnormalities localized to frontotemporal and anterior regions than patients who had not been abused.

Table 9–1. Prevalance of abnormalities on neurological assessment

Abuse history	Neuroimaging study	Neurological exam	Neuropsychological testing	Electrophysiological assessment
None	15.0% (3/20)	50.0% (13/26)	88.0% (22/25)	26.9% (7/26)
Any abuse	26.0% (13/50)	55.4% (41/74)	87.5% (56/64)	54.4% (37/68)
Significance	NS	NS	NS	.021
Psychological	35.7% (5/14)	50.0% (10/20)	78.9% (15/19)	42.9% (9/21)
Physical/sexual (all probable cases)	22.2% (8/36)	57.4% (31/54)	91.1% (41/45)	59.6% (28/47)*
Physical/sexual (only definite serious cases)	23.1% (6/26)	57.9% (22/38)	93.9% (31/33)	71.9% (23/32)**

Note. NS = not significant. *P = .014 versus nonabused. **P = .0013 versus nonabused.

Table 9–2. Prevalance of abnormal electrophysiological findings by age group and gender

Group	Prevalance
Nonabused	26.9% (7/26)
Any abuse	
Men	55.6% (15/27)
Children	56.3% (9/16)
Adolescents	54.5% (6/11)
Women	53.7% (22/41)
Children	53.3% (8/15)
Adolescents	53.8% (14/26)

Table 9–3. Regional localization of electrophysiological abnormalities

Abuse history	Frontotemporal and anterior	Frontal	Temporal
None	19.2% (5/26)	7.7% (2/26)	15.4% (4/26)
Any abuse	47.1% (32/68)	25.0% (17/68)	32.4% (22/68)
Significance	.018	.085	.126
Psychological	38.1% (8/21)	14.3% (3/21)	28.6% (6/21)
Physical/sexual (all probable cases)	51.1% (24/47)**	29.8% (14/47)*	34.0% (16/47)
Physical/sexual (only definite serious cases)	59.4% (19/32)***	37.5% (12/32)**	34.4% (11/32)

*$P = .038$ versus nonabused. **$P = .012$ versus nonabused. ***$P = .0027$ versus nonabused.

As seen in Table 9–4, abused and nonabused patients differed most clearly in the prevalence of left-sided frontotemporal abnormalities ($P = .036$). They did not differ in the prevalence either of right-sided abnormalities ($P > .8$) or of abnormalities that were

Table 9–4. Left-right localization of frontotemporal and anterior electrophysiological abnormalities

Abuse history	Left	Unlocalized or bilateral	Right	Left/right ratio
None	3.8% (1/26)	7.7% (2/26)	7.7% (2/26)	0.50
Any abuse Significance	22.1% (15/68) .036	16.2% (11/68) NS	8.8% (6/68) NS	2.50
Psychological	23.8% (5/21)*	14.3% (3/21)	0.0% (0/21)	∅
Physical/sexual (all probable cases)	21.3% (10/47)*	17.0% (8/47)	12.8% (6/47)	1.67
Physical/sexual (only definite serious cases)	18.8% (6/32)	25.0% (8/32)	15.6% (5/32)	1.20

Note. NS = not significant. *$P = .10$ versus nonabused.

seen bilaterally or that were not specifically localized ($P = .5$). In the nonabused group, left-sided electrophysiological abnormalities were rare. In the abused group, left-sided abnormalities were 2.5-fold more prevalent than right-sided abnormalities. This was particularly true in the psychologically abused group: left-sided electrophysiological abnormalities were present in five cases and right-sided abnormalities were present in none. Furthermore, all of the left-sided abnormalities in the psychological abuse group were restricted to the temporal lobes. It thus appeared that although the overall incidence of electrophysiological abnormalities was numerically, but not statistically, increased in the psychologically abused group, there was a trend for a specific increase in the prevalence of left-sided temporal abnormalities. In the physical/sexual abuse group, there was an overall increase in the prevalence of frontotemporal abnormalities, with less evidence for left-sided localization, particularly in the subgroup with a history of unequivocal serious abuse.

To further explore the possibility that psychological abuse may affect the development of the left hemisphere, the results of neuropsychological testing were reviewed for evidence of right–left hemispheric asymmetries (i.e., substantially better visuospatial ability than verbal performance). Overall, in the nonabused group, left hemisphere deficits were 2.25-fold more prevalent than right hemisphere deficits. In the total abuse group, left-sided deficits were 6.67-fold more prevalent than right, and left hemisphere deficits were 8-fold more prevalent than right-sided deficits in patients with a history of psychological abuse. Thus, abuse appears to be associated with an increased prevalence of both left-sided EEG abnormalities and right–left hemispheric asymmetries.

As in the previous study, there are a number of different ways to interpret a positive association between abuse history and electrophysiological abnormalities. Davies (1978–1979) had suggested that EEG abnormalities may constitute a risk factor for being abused, leading to a higher rate of victimization. It is also conceivable that EEG abnormalities may be inherited; thus, similar abnormalities may be present in parents or siblings and may then be associated with a greater incidence of abusive behavior on the part of these nuclear relatives of the patient. We propose that EEG abnormalities may, however, be a *consequence* of early abuse. However, in order to establish a causal relationship, it will be necessary to conduct a prospective, longitudinal assessment study.

It is also worth pondering what it may mean that psychological abuse seemed to be most strongly associated with left hemisphere abnormalities. Research reviewed above suggests that the right hemisphere may be specialized for the processing of emotion, particularly negative emotions (see also Ahern and Schwartz 1985; Ladavas et al. 1984; Schwartz et al. 1975). Galin (1974) and Joseph (1988) further speculated that painful childhood memories may be preferentially stored in the right hemisphere, outside of consciousness yet capable of influencing conscious behavior and affect. The present findings suggest that childhood abuse may be associated with greater left-sided dysfunction, which may lead to greater dependence on the right hemisphere. Increased right frontal function, in turn, may lead to enhanced perception and reaction to negative affect (Tomarken et al. 1992) and may facilitate unconscious storage of painful childhood memories (Joseph 1988). While this reasoning is merely speculation, it is consistent with the clinical observation that traumatized individuals are often hypersensitive to perception of negative affect and that memories of early abuse may be fully repressed, but eventually retrievable. Muller (1992), in a provocative article, has argued that early difficulties in maternal-child interaction may foster poor integration in right–left hemispheric function and produce a necessary or sufficient neural substrate for borderline splitting.

Right/Left Evoked Response Asymmetry During Recall of Unpleasant Early Memories in Psychologically Traumatized Subjects

Schiffer and colleagues (F. Schiffer, M. H. Teicher, and A. C. Papanicolaou, November 1993 [unpublished manuscript]) have used probe auditory evoked potential attenuation as a measure of hemispheric activity to further study the effects of early trauma on cerebral laterality. As stated previously, Galin (1974) and Joseph (1988) postulated that painful childhood memories might be preferentially stored in the right hemisphere, from which they might influence conscious behavior and affect. To further evaluate this hypothesis, hemispheric brain activity was measured in adult subjects under two conditions: 1) during recall of a neutral work-related situation and 2) during recall of an unpleasant affectively laden early memory. Probe auditory evoked potentials (AEPs) were used as an index of hemispheric activity. Subjects were exposed to repeated auditory clicks while the amplitude of the average evoked potential EEG response was measured. While exposed to the clicks, the subjects were asked to engage in a mental activity. When one hemisphere is more actively involved than the other, the AEP response is attenuated in that hemisphere (Papanicolaou and Johnstone 1984; Papanicolaou et al. 1983a, 1983b). AEPs were studied in 10 right-handed adult subjects, all of whom were psychotropic free. The subjects were first asked to remember and reflect on an ordinary work or school situation. AEPs were recorded after the subjects indicated that they were actively remembering the situation. Following the recording, the subjects were given a number of queries taken from the Profile of Mood States (POMS; Lorr et al. 1971). Each subject was then engaged in an empathic psychiatric interview lasting about 15 minutes. The psychiatrist tried to affectively engage the subject and to have him or her share, with emotion, a painful childhood memory. When it was felt that the subject was affectively reexperiencing the memory, the psychiatrist asked him or her to try to continue to maintain the memory without speech or motion so that AEPs could be measured. Following recording, the POMS was used again to measure the subject's emotional state. All results from AEP recordings were scored blindly by a research electrophysiologist.

Of the 10 subjects studied, 5 had experienced extreme psychological trauma during childhood, 2 had experienced severe trauma, 2 had experienced moderate trauma, and 1 had experienced no significant trauma. Overall, the neutral memory task produced a low mood score that was increased by about 8-fold during recall of the early abusive memory. Specifically, recall of the early abusive memories resulted in substantially increased levels of tension, anger, sadness, hopelessness, nervousness, and panic.

During the neutral task, eight subjects had higher amplitudes over the right auditory cortex than the left, implying greater relative left-sided cortical activity (left-sided attenuation). During recall of the unpleasant memory, seven subjects had lower amplitudes over the right auditory cortex than the left, implying greater relative right-sided cortical activity (right-sided attenuation) ($P < .02$). Moreover, there was a significant correlation between ratings of severity of early psychiatric trauma and blind assessment of the degree of shift in the asymmetry index between tasks (Spearman's $\rho = .586$, $P < .05$).

These findings are consistent with a large number of studies that demonstrate increased right hemisphere involvement with a number of affective tasks. Of particular interest was the observation that the degree of left–right shift correlated with estimates of the severity of the subject's early abuse. This observation suggests that early traumatic experiences may play a role in fostering the specialization of the right hemisphere or in preventing the development of greater hemispheric interconnectivity. Unfortunately, it is not possible to distinguish between the possibility that the right hemisphere is merely specialized to handle emotions and the more intriguing hypothesis that early abusive memories may be stored in the right hemisphere outside of conscious awareness. In any case, these findings are consistent with a hypothesis that childhood trauma influences hemispheric laterality. One could speculate that increased right hemispheric dominance may contribute to a more affectively laden, negative perception of the world (Tomarken et al. 1992), which may be part of the problem in certain patients with BPD (Baker et al. 1992; Nigg et al. 1991).

SUMMARY AND CONCLUSIONS

The studies presented here support our initial hypothesis that early abuse may be associated with features of limbic system dysfunction, EEG abnormalities, and measures of hemispheric asymmetry. However, these studies do not provide strong proof, which would require prospective demonstration of the emergence of electrophysiological abnormalities or hemispheric asymmetries in previously normal children after the occurrence of early abuse. Obviously, such a study would be logistically and ethically difficult.

In addition, these studies lend additional support to previous observations that a significant association exists between childhood abuse and evidence of neurobiological abnormalities. We cannot, however, disentangle the hypothesis that early abuse may lead to neurobiological abnormalities from the equally plausible hypothesis that the presence of neurobiological abnormalities may increase the risk of childhood abuse. Regardless of the direction, the nature of the association indicates that in order to obtain a complete understanding of the causes, consequences, treatment, and prevention of childhood abuse, an integrated biopsychosocial model is necessary.

Our specific hypothesis is that early abuse can lead to a variety of neurodevelopmental abnormalities with different behavioral sequelae. Influencing neuroadrenergic inputs to the hippocampus can result in anxiogenic, amnestic, somatic, and dissociative effects. Kindled foci in the amygdala or serotonin deficiencies in the septo-hippocampal behavioral inhibitory system can lead to the inappropriate release of aggressive and sexual behavior; irritability can result from similar disinhibitory influences in the prefrontal cortex. Deficient integration of left and right hemisphere function may result in the misperception of affect and thereby foster a situation in which the right and left halves of the brain act uncooperatively. Lack of appropriate hemispheric interdependence may give rise to intrapsychic conflict or create affective instability if the right hemisphere floods the left with emotions and moods that do not make logical sense.

If the model we propose is valid, then the consequences of abuse would depend on the age at onset, duration, and severity of the trauma, because different regions would have different windows or thresholds of vulnerability. One possible prediction of this model is that psychotherapy and somatic treatment during adulthood may be insufficient to correct the effects of early abuse if such abuse results in irreversible structural neurological abnormalities. It is even conceivable that attempting to recall the abuse and "work through the trauma" could lead to temporary or persistent worsening of symptoms if such attempts further exacerbate kindling. While this last point is merely theoretical speculation and should in no way influence our clinical practice, it is probably fair to suggest that greater attention should be given to the prevention of abuse or to early therapeutic interventions as potentially cost-effective alternatives. Although additional research is certainly necessary to establish a link between early abuse, limbic system dysfunction, and the genesis of borderline personality, it is our hope that this model will stimulate research and thoughtful discussion.

REFERENCES

Ahern GL, Schwartz GE: Differential lateralization for positive and negative emotion in the human brain: EEG spectral analysis. Neuropsychologia 23:745–756, 1985

Alexander GE, Goldman PS: Functional development of the dorsolateral prefrontal cortex: an analysis utilizing reversible cryogenic depression. Brain Res 143:233–249, 1978

Andrulonis PA, Glueck BC, Stroebel CF, et al: Organic brain dysfunction and the borderline syndrome. Psychiatr Clin North Am 4:47–66, 1981

Bach-y-Rita G, Lion JR, Climent CE, et al: Episodic dyscontrol: a study of 130 violent patients. Am J Psychiatry 127:1473–1478, 1971

Baker L, Silk KR, Westen D, et al: Malevolence, splitting, and parental ratings by borderlines. J Nerv Ment Dis 180:258–264, 1992

Beck JC, van der Kolk B: Reports of childhood incest and current behavior of chronically hospitalized psychotic women. Am J Psychiatry 144:1474–1476, 1987

Bernstein EM, Putnam FW: Development, reliability and validity of a dissociation scale. J Nerv Ment Dis 174:727–735, 1986

Bliss EL: Multiple personalities: a report of 14 cases with implications for schizophrenia and hysteria. Arch Gen Psychiatry 37:1388–1397, 1980

Borod JC: Interhemispheric and intrahemispheric control of emotion: a focus on unilateral brain damage. J Consult Clin Psychol 60:339–348, 1992

Brende JO: The psychophysiologic manifestations of dissociation: electrodermal responses in a multiple personality patient. Psychiatr Clin North Am 7:41–49, 1984

Bryer JB, Nelson BA, Miller JB, et al: Childhood sexual and physical abuse as factors in adult psychiatric illness. Am J Psychiatry 144:1426–1430, 1987

Burgess AW, Hartmann CR, McCormack A: Abused to abuser: antecedents of socially deviant behavior. Am J Psychiatry 144:1431–1436, 1987

Burgess JW: Neurocognitive impairment in dramatic personalities: histrionic, narcissistic, borderline, and antisocial disorders. Psychiatry Res 42:283–90, 1992

Coccaro EF, Siever LJ, Klar HM, et al: Serotonergic studies in patients with affective and personality disorders: correlates with suicidal and impulsive aggressive behavior. Arch Gen Psychiatry 46:587–599, 1989

Coons PM, Bowman ES, Milstein V: Multiple personality disorder: a clinical investigation of 50 cases. J Nerv Ment Dis 176:519–527, 1988

Cornelius JR, Brenner RP, Soloff PH, et al: EEG abnormalities in borderline personality disorder: specific or nonspecific. Biol Psychiatry 21:974–977, 1986

Cornelius JR, Schulz SC, Brenner RP, et al: Changes in EEG mean frequency associated with anxiety and with amphetamine challenge in BPD. Biol Psychiatry 24:587–594, 1988

Cowdry RW, Pickar D, Davies R: Symptoms and EEG findings in the borderline syndrome. Int J Psychiatry Med 15:201–211, 1985–1986

Cynader M, Lepore F, Guillemot JP: Inter-hemispheric competition during postnatal development. Nature 290:139–140, 1981

Davidson R, Ekman P, Saron CD, et al: Approach-withdrawal and cerebral asymmetry: emotional expression and brain physiology. J Pers Soc Psychol 58:330–341, 1990

Davies RK: Incest: some neuropsychiatric findings. Int J Psychiatry Med 9:117–121, 1978–1979

Denenberg VH: Lateralization of function in rats. Am J Physiol 245:R505–R509, 1983

Depue RA, Spoont MR: Conceptualizing a serotonin trait: a behavioral dimension of constraint. Ann N Y Acad Sci 487:47–62, 1986

Derogatis LR, Lipman RS, Rickels K, et al: The Hopkins Symptom Checklist (HSCL): a self-report symptom inventory. Behav Sci 19:1–15, 1974

Deutch AY, Tam S-Y, Roth RH: Footshock and conditioned stress increase 3,4-dihydroxyphenylacetic acid (DOPAC) in the ventral tegmental area but not substantia nigra. Brain Res 333:143–146, 1985

Domesick VB: Neuroanatomical organization of the dopamine neurons in the ventral tegmental area. Ann N Y Acad Sci 537:10–26, 1988

Famularo R, Kinscherff R, Fenton T: Propranolol treatment for childhood posttraumatic stress disorder, acute type: a pilot study. Am J Dis Child 142:1244–1247, 1988

Faravelli C, Webb T, Ambonetti A: Prevalence of traumatic early life events in 31 agoraphobic patients with panic attacks. Am J Psychiatry 142:1493–1494, 1985

Finkelhor D: A Sourcebook on Child Sexual Abuse. Beverly Hills, CA, Sage, 1986

Fox NA, Davidson RJ: Taste-elicited changes in facial signs of emotion and the asymmetry of brain electrical activity in human newborns. Neuropsychologia 24:417–22, 1986

Fuster JM: The Prefrontal Cortex: Anatomy, Physiology, and Neuropsychology of the Frontal Lobe. New York, Raven, 1980

Galin D: Implications for psychiatry of left and right cerebral specialization. Arch Gen Psychiatry 31:572–583, 1974

Galin D: Lateral specialization and psychiatric issues: speculations on development and the evolution of consciousness. Ann N Y Acad Sci 299:397–411, 1977

Goddard GV, Mcintyre DC, Leech CK: A permanent change in brain functioning resulting from daily electrical stimulation. Exp Neurol 25:295–330, 1969

Goodin DS, Aminoff MJ: Does the interictal EEG have a role in the diagnosis of epilepsy? Lancet 1(8381):837–839, 1984

Goldman PS: Functional development of the prefrontal cortex in early life and the problem of neuronal plasticity. Exp Neurol 32:366–387, 1971

Gorman JM, Liebowitz MR, Fryer AJ, et al: A neuroanatomical hypothesis for panic disorder. Am J Psychiatry 146:148–161, 1989

Gray JA, Holt L, McNaughton N: Clinical implications of the experimental pharmacology of the benzodiazepines, in The Benzodiazepines: From Molecular Biology to Clinical Practice. Edited by Costa E. New York, Raven, 1983, pp 147–171

Green AH: Dimensions of psychological trauma in abused children. Journal of the American Academy of Child Psychiatry 22:231–237, 1983

Green AH, Voeller K, Gaines R, et al: Neurological impairment in maltreated children. Child Abuse Negl 5:129–134, 1981

Herman JL: Histories of violence in an outpatient population. Am J Orthopsychiatry 56:137–141, 1986

Herman JL, Perry JC, van der Kolk BA: Childhood trauma in borderline personality disorder. Am J Psychiatry 146:490–495, 1989

Hirschman RS, Safer MA: Hemispheric differences in perceiving positive and negative emotions. Cortex 18:569–580, 1982

Hofer MA: Studies on how early maternal separation produces behavioral change in young rats. Psychosom Med 37:245–264, 1975

Horevitz RP, Braun BR: Are multiple personalities borderlines? An analysis of 33 cases. Psychiatr Clin North Am 7:69–87, 1984

Hubel DH: Effects of deprivation on the visual cortex of cat and monkey. Harvey Lectures 72:1–51, 1978

Ito Y, Teicher MH, Glod CA, et al: Increased prevalence of electrophysiological abnormalities in children with psychological, physical, and sexual abuse. J Neuropsychiatry Clin Neurosci 5:401–408, 1993

Joseph R: The right cerebral hemisphere: emotion, music, visual-spatial skills, body-image, dreams, and awareness. J Clin Psychol 44:630–673, 1988

Kashani JH, Carlson GA: Seriously depressed preschoolers. Am J Psychiatry 144:348–350, 1987

Knorr AM, Deutch AY, Roth RH: The anxiogenic-carboline FG-7142 increases in vivo and in vitro tyrosine hydroxylation in the prefrontal cortex. Brain Res 495:355–361, 1989

Krystal H: Trauma and affects. Psychoanal Study Child 33:81–116, 1978

Ladavas E, Nicoletti R, Umlita C, et al: Right hemisphere interference during negative affect: a reaction time study. Neuropsychologia 22:479–485, 1984

Levitt P: A monoclonal antibody to limbic system neurons. Science 223:299–301, 1984

Links PS, Steiner M, Offord DR, et al: Characteristics of borderline personality disorder: a Canadian study. Can J Psychiatry 33:336–340, 1988

Lopes da Silva FH, Witter MP, Boeijinga PH, et al: Anatomic organization and physiology of the limbic cortex. Physiol Rev 70:453–511 1990

Lorr M, McNair DM, Droppleman LF: Manual: Profile of Mood States. San Diego, CA, Educational and Industrial Testing Service, 1971

Matthews WB: The use and abuse of electroencephalography. Lancet 2:577–579, 1964

Mesulam MM: Dissociative states with abnormal temporal lobe EEG: multiple personality and the illusion of possession. Arch Neurol 38:176–181, 1981

Muller RJ: Is there a neural basis for borderline splitting? Compr Psychiatry 33:92–104, 1992

Nigg JT, Silk KR, Westen D, et al: Object representations in the early memories of sexually abused borderline patients. Am J Psychiatry 148:864–869, 1991

Ogata SN, Silk KR, Goodrich S, et al: Childhood sexual and physical abuse in adult patients with borderline personality disorder. Am J Psychiatry 147:1008–1013, 1990

O'Leary KM, Brouwers P, Gardner DL, et al: Neuropsychological testing of patients with borderline personality disorder. Am J Psychiatry 148:106–111, 1991

Papanicolaou AC, Johnstone J: Probe evoked potentials: theory, method and applications. Int J Neurosci 24:107–131 1984

Papanicolaou AC, Schmidt AL, Moore BD, et al: Cerebral activation patterns in an arithmetic and a visuospatial processing task. Int J Neurosci 20:283–287, 1983a

Papanicolaou AC, Levin HS, Eisenberg HM, et al: Evoked potential indices of selective hemispheric engagement in affective and phonetic tasks. Neuropsychologia 21:401–405, 1983b

Pincus JH, Tucker GJ: Behavioral Neurology. New York, Oxford University Press, 1978, pp 58–79

Post RM, Rubinow DR, Ballenger JC: Conditioning, sensitization, and kindling: implications for the course of affective illness, in Neurobiology of Mood Disorders. Edited by Post RM, Ballenger JC. Baltimore, MD, Williams & Wilkins, 1984, pp 432–466

Putnam FW, Guroff JJ, Silverman EK, et al: The clinical phenomenology of multiple personality disorder: review of 100 recent cases. J Clin Psychiatry 47:285–293, 1986

Reep R: Relationship between prefrontal and limbic cortex: a comparative anatomical review. Brain Behav Evol 25:5–80, 1984

Reiman EM, Raichle ME, Butler FK, et al: A focal brain abnormality in panic disorder, a severe form of anxiety. Nature 310:683–685, 1984

Reinhard JF Jr, Bannon MJ, Roth RH: Acceleration by stress of dopamine synthesis and metabolism in prefrontal cortex: antagonism by diazepam. Naunyn-Schmiedebergs Arch Pharmacol 318:374–377, 1982

Ross CA, Heber S, Anderson G, et al: Differentiating multiple personality disorder and complex partial seizures. Gen Hosp Psychiatry 11:54–58, 1989

Ross ED: The aprosodias: functional-anatomic organization of the affective components of language in the right hemisphere. Arch Neurol 38:561–569, 1981

Sapolsky RM, Uno H, Rebert CS, et al: Hippocampal damage associated with prolonged glucocorticoid exposure in primates. J Neurosci 10:2897–2902, 1990

Schenk L, Baer D: Multiple personality and related dissociative phenomenon in patients with temporal lobe epilepsy. Am J Psychiatry 138:1311–1316, 1981

Schwartz GE, Davidson RJ, Maer F: Right hemisphere lateralization for emotion in the human brain: interaction with cognition. Science 190:286–288, 1975

Shearer SL, Peters CP, Quaytman MS, et al: Frequency and correlates of childhood sexual and physical abuse histories in adult female borderline inpatients. Am J Psychiatry 147:214–216, 1990

Silberman EK, Weingartner H: Hemispheric lateralization of functions related to emotion. Brain Cogn 5:322–353, 1986

Snyder S, Pitts WM Jr: Electroencephalograph of DSM-III borderline personality disorder. Acta Psychiatr Scand 69:129–134, 1984

Spiers PA, Schomer DL, Blume HW, et al: Temporolimbic epilepsy and behavior, in Principles of Behavioral Neurology. Edited by Mesulam MM. Philadelphia, PA, FA Davis, 1985, pp 289–326

Stone MH: Borderline syndromes: a consideration of subtypes and an overview, directions for research. Psychiatr Clin North Am 4:3–13, 1981

Struve FA, Klein DF, Saraf KR: Electroencephalographic correlates of suicide ideation and attempts. Arch Gen Psychiatry 27:363–365, 1972

Teicher MH: Biology of anxiety. Med Clin N Am 72:791–814, 1988

Teicher MH: Psychological factors in neurological development, in Neurobiological Development (Nestle Nutrition Workshop Series, Vol 12). Edited by Evrard P, Minkowski A. New York, Raven, 1989, pp 243–258

Teicher MH, Glod CA, Surrey J, et al: Childhood abuse and limbic system ratings in adult psychiatric outpatients. J Neuropsychiatry Clin Neurosci 5:301–306, 1993

Tomarken AJ, Davidson RJ, Wheeler RE, et al: Individual differences in anterior brain asymmetry and fundamental dimensions of emotion. J Pers Soc Psychol 62:676–687, 1992

van der Kolk BA, Greenberg MS: The psychobiology of the trauma response: hyperarousal, constriction, and addiction to traumatic reexposure, in Psychological Trauma. Edited by van der Kolk BA. Washington, DC, American Psychiatric Press, 1987, pp 63–87

Weinberger DR: Implications of normal brain development for the pathogenesis of schizophrenia. Arch Gen Psychiatry 44:660–669, 1987

Westen D, Ludolph P, Misle B, et al: Physical and sexual abuse in adolescent girls with borderline personality disorder. Am J Orthopsychiatry 60:55–66, 1990

Zanarini MC, Gunderson JG, Marino MF, et al: Childhood experiences of borderline patients. Compr Psychiatry 30:18–25, 1989

Chapter 10

"Quo Vademus?"— New Directions in Borderline Personality Disorder Research

Rex William Cowdry, M.D.

The complexities of the human brain and mind have not yielded easily to the reductionism inherent in the scientific method. The difficulties in developing comprehensive scientific theories about the etiology of major mental illnesses are evident from the succession of conflicting theories that have been put forth during this century. Schizophrenia, to choose a particularly dramatic example, has been explained by a series of theories proposing neurological, developmental, psychosocial, neurochemical, neurodevelopmental, and infectious causes and implicating abnormal genes, faulty parenting, faulty ontogeny, abnormal neurotransmission, viruses, and other factors. Evidence of a substantial biological component in the etiology of schizophrenia is incontrovertible, yet no single biological abnormality is found universally in schizophrenic patients. Evidence for a substantial hereditary component is also incontrovertible, but the existence of discordant identical twins suggests that heredity alone cannot explain the disorder.

Theories of personality disorders have undergone similar transitions in the 20th century. Beginning with a strong focus on constitutional factors such as heredity and electroencephalogram (EEG) abnormalities, theories of personality progressed through a period that emphasized early development and psychosocial influences and moved into a second era of phenomenological, behavioral, and biological investigations.

This rekindling of interest in the phenomenology and behavioral biology of personality disorders has been fueled by several developments. On the one hand, developmental and psychosocial theories have not adequately explained personality disorders and have not produced particularly useful interventions. On the other hand, recent dramatic advances in basic and animal research have led to breakthroughs in our understanding of brain function, and new clinical research techniques using pharmacological probes and structural and functional brain imaging have produced a literal and figurative depth of investigation heretofore impossible.

The current generation of biologically and behaviorally oriented research studies reflects the excitement accompanying this latest swing of the pendulum. Contemporary research efforts are likely to lead to three outcomes: 1) biological underpinnings will be identified for many personality disorders, thereby leading to more effective interventions; 2) the limitations of purely biological explanations will become clearer; and 3) theories of personality and its disorders will increasingly emphasize interactions between biology and experience.

The chapters in this volume provide an excellent introduction to contemporary trends in borderline personality disorder (BPD) research. These chapters represent attempts to conceptualize current approaches to personality disorder research, to identify the advantages and possible shortcomings of each approach, and to place these individual approaches in context.

APPROACHES TO BORDERLINE PERSONALITY DISORDER THROUGH ANALOGY TO AXIS I DISORDERS

One prominent approach to BPD has been to regard aspects of the disorder as analogous to aspects of the more heavily researched Axis I disorders. Siever and Davis (1991) have summarized well the arguments for regarding the prominent features of personality disorders in general and BPD in particular as variants of similar dimensions of behavior among the Axis I affective, schizophrenic, or impulsive spectrum disorders. In contrast to the origin of the term *borderline* in earlier American concepts of schizophrenia, BPD itself does not appear to be related to schizophrenia proper, although family and twin studies have suggested that schizotypal personality disorder (which may coexist with BPD) may be part of a broadly defined spectrum of schizophreniform disorders (see, e.g., Kendler et al. 1981). Concurrent affective disorder, particularly major depression but possibly bipolar mood disorder as well, is common in BPD, but the relationship between the affective disorders and BPD is far from clear, as reviewed by Gunderson and Phillips (1991).

Early biological studies of BPD attempted to document possible relationships of BPD to Axis I disorders by borrowing the biological techniques applied to Axis I disorders. With regard to the interface of BPD with the schizophrenias, individuals with schizotypal personality disorder appear to have an increased prevalence of the smooth-pursuit eye movement abnormalities found in schizophrenia (Siever 1985). With regard to the interface with the affective disorders, neuroendocrine challenges, such as the dexamethasone suppression test and the thyrotropin-releasing hormone (TRH) test, and sleep architecture studies (Akiskal et al. 1985; McNamara et al. 1984) have demonstrated an increased prevalence of abnormalities in BPD. These abnormal findings were originally interpreted as indications of a relationship between mood disorders and BPD, but they may instead be a reflection of the diagnostic nonspecificity of such biological disturbances (Siever et al. 1985).

Analogies to Axis I disorders are extremely useful insofar as they may stimulate research into biological similarities underlying the phenomenological similarities and eventually lead to new treatment approaches. However, research using analogies to Axis I disorders must address the limitations of these analogies. Phenomenological dissimilarities should be identified. For example, although BPD may involve mood states much like the extremes of bipolar illness, the temporal pattern of the mood changes is more random, the mood shifts more frequent, the reactivity of the mood to specific stressors (loss or rejection) more prominent, and the autonomy of the mood state less evident. There are also dissimilarities in pharmacological response that must be addressed. For example, why do symptoms in BPD respond (at least in part) to much lower dosages of neuroleptics than Axis I psychoses and (perhaps more importantly) why do they generally respond rapidly rather than over a period of weeks? Finally, for Axis I analogies to be useful, they must usefully guide treatment. At this point in time, the clinical implications of phenomenological and biological similarities between Axis I and Axis II disorders are unclear. Do these Axis I/Axis II similarities predict medication response, episode outcome, or longitudinal course within the borderline population?

NEW BORDERS FOR BORDERLINE PERSONALITY DISORDER

Panic and Anxiety Disorders

As described by Silk et al. in Chapter 5, the acute episodes of anxiety and dysphoria seen in BPD have strong phenomenological similarities to panic attacks. Clinically, it is not uncommon to encounter individuals with BPD who describe their episodes as panic-laden and who sometimes specifically seek evaluation and treatment in an anxiety disorder program. Phenomenological similarities between the panic/anxiety disorders and BPD as well as possible biological underpinnings in the adrenergic or cholinergic systems are the subject of the chapters by Steinberg et al. (Chapter 3), Yehuda et al. (Chapter 4), and Silk et al. (Chapter 5).

Trauma, Posttraumatic Stress Disorder, and Multiple Personality Disorder

Over the past decade, it has become increasingly evident that trauma in general, and physical or sexual abuse in particular, are general risk factors for psychiatric disorders, have a direct causal relationship to posttraumatic stress disorder (PTSD) (although other vulnerability factors may play an important role), and are strongly associated with multiple personality disorder (MPD). The prevalence of physical and sexual abuse histories among BPD patients is also high (Herman et al. 1989; Ogata et al. 1990;

Westen et al. 1990; Zanarini et al. 1989). A number of theorists have come to regard BPD as a form of PTSD, but with the psychological trauma occurring at a different developmental stage. Gunderson and Sabo's (1993) recent review of the relationship of PTSD to BPD provides a thorough discussion of the similarities and dissimilarities of these disorders. It remains unclear whether treatment strategies applied to PTSD can be adapted as primary treatments for BPD. From a biological perspective, research into biological vulnerability factors and pharmacological interventions in PTSD may have some relevance to the biology and pharmacotherapy of BPD.

The relationship of BPD to MPD is also of particular interest. A substantial number of MPD patients meet criteria for BPD as well, particularly when MPD patients demonstrate prominent affective lability and periods of behavioral dyscontrol. Dissociative symptoms are, of course, fundamental features of MPD, but dissociative symptoms are also very common in BPD (Silk et al. 1989; Zweig-Frank et al. 1993). Do both disorders have a common origin in dissociative defense mechanisms in response to trauma? Is the affective lability of BPD in part a product of state changes associated with dissociation, as in MPD? At present, these questions cannot be answered with any degree of confidence.

Behavioral and Cognitive Dyscontrol

BPD also demonstrates both phenomenological overlap and diagnostic comorbidity with other disorders characterized by behavioral or cognitive dyscontrol. The rage episodes and violent behavior in BPD (and the underlying failure to bind primitive affect with thought) resemble behavior in explosive disorders. Eating disorders and BPD show substantial comorbidity. Ruminative behavior, particularly obsessional concern with suicidal thoughts, has a repetitive, "uncontrollable" quality similar to that seen in other obsessional disorders (although the repetitive thinking is usually more ego-syntonic than that seen in classical obsessive-compulsive disorder). As biological underpinnings of such impulsive, ruminative, or repetitive behaviors have been identified and specific pharmacological interventions found to be at least partially effective, researchers and clinicians have tried to determine both the relevance of these mechanisms to BPD and the effectiveness of these treatments in BPD.

The relationship between BPD and substance abuse has not been well delineated beyond the greater-than-chance comorbidity. Even the direction of postulated causal links are controversial. Do both disorders arise from deficits in executive functions? Does substance abuse contribute substantially to the observed affective and behavioral dysregulation? Is substance abuse an attempt to self-medicate to relieve depression, anxiety, rage, or dysphoria?

THE RISE OF DIMENSIONAL APPROACHES AND THEIR POSSIBLE BIOLOGICAL UNDERPINNINGS

Biologically oriented research in the personality disorders increasingly employs dimensional approaches to psychopathology. These dimensional approaches in biological research are in contrast to the categorical approaches used by current diagnostic schemata. (For examples of dimensional approaches, see Cloninger [1987] and Widiger et al. [1987].) Specific dimensions of psychopathology are postulated to have a common biological underpinning across disorders, and research is directed toward the identification of biological correlates of psychopathological dimensions and dimensional symptom responses to pharmacological treatment interventions.

Impulsivity

The most widely researched dimension, which extends across Axis I as well as Axis II disorders, is the dimension variously characterized as behavioral dyscontrol, impulsivity, aggression, violence, and suicidal or self-injurious behavior. This dimension is reviewed and discussed by deVegvar et al. in Chapter 2. In Chapter 1, van Reekum et al. explore some of the nosological difficulties in defining the term *impulsivity*. The link between this dimension and the serotonergic system in particular has its roots in animal research and has become one of the best-established clinical-biological correlates. Researchers have assessed serotonergic function in vitro through postmortem studies of the brain and in vivo through studies of the serotonin metabolite 5-hydroxyindoleacetic acid (5-HIAA) in cerebrospinal fluid, through neuroendocrine challenges with serotonergic agents, and through direct serum assays and platelet receptor assays. Coccaro et al. (1990) have thoroughly reviewed the research regarding the role of serotonin in personality disorders. A natural outgrowth of this biological research is the current pharmacological study of the efficacy of selective serotonin reuptake inhibitors in these behavioral syndromes.

Affective Instability

Affective instability constitutes another symptom dimension that is prominent in BPD but that has proven harder to research, both biologically and pharmacologically. Steinberg et al. review this issue in Chapter 3. BPD tends to be characterized by rapid, environmentally responsive mood shifts—most commonly, the development of rage, anxiety, depression, and/or dysphoria in response to perceived loss or rejection. Although certain pharmacological challenges (e.g., intravenous procaine [Kellner et al. 1987] or methylphenidate [Lucas et al. 1987]) appear capable of evoking dysphoric states in BPD, the specificity of the response and the underlying biological mechanism is far from clear.

Central Nervous System Dysfunction

Central nervous system (CNS) dysfunction, particularly dysfunction in the limbic system, has been postulated to underlie a variety of behaviors prominent in BPD. In Chapter 9, Teicher et al. consider an intriguing theory that links limbic system dysfunction and trauma to explain much borderline behavior. Episodic dyscontrol as described by Monroe (1970) has features in common with the behavioral dyscontrol so prominent in BPD. Symptoms often observed in complex partial seizures (absence episodes, depersonalization, derealization, and déjà vu, among others) are frequently found in patients with BPD (although these symptoms are also prominent in dissociative syndromes secondary to physical or sexual abuse). In one double-blind study, carbamazepine was shown to significantly decrease the frequency and severity of behavioral dyscontrol in BPD (Gardner and Cowdry 1986). Various authors have suggested that a number of clinical aspects of BPD are consistent with epileptoid phenomena in limbic structures. The possibility of CNS dysfunction has also been raised in the context of attention-deficit disorder (ADD). ADD in adulthood appears to be characterized by affective lability and behavioral impulsivity, and a high prevalence of childhood ADD was found in males in one study of adolescents with BPD (Andrulonis et al. 1981). However, concrete evidence of specific or consistent CNS abnormalities or dysfunction in BPD has not been found. Gross CNS pathology has not been demonstrated in several structural imaging studies of BPD (Lucas et al. 1989; Snyder et al. 1983). Imaging studies in BPD are described in more detail in Chapter 6 by Goyer et al. Routine EEG studies with borderline patients have found only nonspecific and inconsistent EEG abnormalities (Cowdry et al. 1985–1986; Snyder and Pitts 1984). Zanarini et al. in Chapter 8 and Teicher et al. in Chapter 9 review current attempts to better appreciate the possible neurological underpinnings of BPD, while in Chapter 7, O'Leary and Cowdry explore neuropsychological test studies as another way to better understand the relationship between BPD and neurological dysfunction.

Self-Mutilation

One of the strangest clinical phenomena associated with BPD is that of repetitive self-mutilation. In half of all episodes, self-mutilation is characterized by anesthesia. Although this anesthesia may reflect the psychological phenomenon of dissociation, one recent research study suggests that individuals reporting anesthesia during self-injury also have high pain thresholds in the cold pressor test under controlled laboratory conditions (Russ et al. 1992). Preliminary reports of abnormal levels of endogenous opiates associated with chronic self-injury in a variety of clinical populations raise the possibility that abnormalities in the endogenous opiate system may be associated with abnormal pain perception (and, conceivably, with anticipatory anhedonia, which is common in BPD). Although research in this area is in its very early stages, it has led to a series of trials of opiate antagonists in the treatment of self-injurious behavior.

Psychosis

The nature and underpinnings of the "psychotic" symptoms of BPD may be distinctive. Zanarini et al. (1990) suggest that the array of psychotic symptoms in BPD can be distinguished from the typical psychotic symptoms of schizophrenia in that the BPD psychotic symptoms tend to resemble dissociative symptoms. As noted in Chapter 5 by Silk and colleagues, some of these episodes also resemble panic attacks. Are these symptoms analogous to other psychotic symptoms and in part dopaminergically mediated? Are they analogous to panic symptoms and in part adrenergically or cholinergically mediated? Or are these symptoms fundamentally dissociative?

THE SPECIAL CONTRIBUTIONS OF THIS VOLUME

Into this ferment come the pioneering research efforts compiled in this book, each with a distinctive perspective on this disorder.

The research on cognitive/neuropsychological abnormalities in BPD, reviewed by O'Leary and Cowdry in Chapter 7, initially appears to be fundamentally descriptive rather than etiological. Although the available studies involve relatively small numbers of subjects and demonstrate some inconsistencies, these studies suggest that cognitive abnormalities (particularly difficulties with complex memory processes and possibly with visuospatial processing) exist in BPD. The presence of cognitive abnormalities per se is hardly a surprise, but the intriguing feature of these cognitive abnormalities is that they appear to be present in relatively affect-neutral situations; that is, these abnormalities may not be a product of intrapsychic conflict and may not serve a defensive function. Such observations tentatively suggest that there is a fundamental cognitive disability in BPD that may reflect an underlying neurophysiological dysfunction.

Two chapters explore more explicitly the possible neurophysiological underpinnings from somewhat different but convergent perspectives. While van Reekum and colleagues have long been interested in the relationship between brain injury and borderline symptoms (van Reekum et al. 1993), in Chapter 1 they turn their attention to trying to understand phenomenologically one of the more common manifestations of brain injury—impulsivity. They conclude that inattentiveness and a tendency toward motor action without anticipation of the consequences may underlie a substantial portion of what is known as impulsivity in BPD. These authors believe that this impulsivity is similar to the impulsivity seen in attention-deficit hyperactivity disorder and in some traumatic brain injuries.

Teicher et al., in Chapter 9, take a more specific correlational approach to linking phenomenological features, developmental trauma, and physiological abnormalities. They define a set of symptoms presumed to originate in the limbic system and assess these symptoms with a structured questionnaire, the Limbic Symptom Checklist—33 (LSCL-33; Teicher et al. 1993). The authors find that these symptoms are associated on the one hand with trauma history and on the other hand with electroencephalographic abnormalities assessed with EEG and brain electrical activity mapping (BEAM) technology. This provocative study raises intriguing issues. Do "limbic symptoms" originate in the limbic system and do these symptoms have some degree of overlap with classical complex partial seizure symptoms and dissociative symptoms? What do the EEG and BEAM assess, and with what specificity? And perhaps most speculatively, a reader might go beyond the data and ask whether some symptoms thought to originate in psychological trauma have a physiological substrate, and if so, how such a substrate develops.

In contrast to these articles, Zanarini et al. (Chapter 8) report a retrospective chart review comparing patients with BPD with patients with other personality disorders (OPD). This review, albeit compromised by the usual limitations of retrospective studies (e.g., incomplete data and selection biases governing which data were available), found no difference between BPD and OPD patients on a variety of clinical indices of neurological dysfunction, although some index of dysfunction was found in a high percentage of both groups. Despite the fact that a significantly higher percentage of BPD than OPD patients reported physical or sexual abuse, there was no association between neurological findings and abuse history. Because diagnostic groups rather than specific dimensions of psychopathology were compared, it is unclear whether the Zanarini et al. study conflicts with Teicher et al.'s study (Chapter 9) or whether clinical elements common to a variety of personality disorders (e.g., impulsivity) have a neurological underpinning that the diagnostic-group-based comparison was unable to identify. Zanarini et al.'s study does suggest an absence of overt neurological sequelae of (or predispositions to) abuse, however, a finding that warrants a definitive prospective study. What is quite intriguing here is that, regardless of diagnosis, sexually abused subjects were referred more frequently for a neurological workup. Despite a lack of significant neurological findings between groups, the question must be asked: What were physicians "picking up" about these patients that prompted them to refer the patients for neurological evaluation?

The dimensional approach to personality disorders is fundamentally an attempt to organize the phenomenology of these disorders into orthogonal symptom dimensions. The resultant symptom dimensions are in turn linked conceptually to biological substrates and, more specifically, to the neurotransmitter systems through which behavioral dimensions are presumed to be regulated.

Yehuda et al., in Chapter 4, present evidence for catecholaminergic dysregulation in BPD. The authors focus primarily on catecholaminergic dysregulation in part because they approach BPD from a different perspective—namely, an assumption that the "near-neighbor" disorder to BPD is PTSD. Research in anxiety, panic, and trauma disorders has demonstrated abnormalities in platelet $alpha_2$-adrenergic receptors and platelet monoamine oxidase (MAO), peripheral adrenergic markers that are presumed to reflect CNS adrenergic states. The presence of demonstrated abnormalities in these peripheral markers strengthens the assumption that the adrenergic system plays a significant role in the expression of symptoms in BPD. Unresolved is the question of whether adrenergic dysregulation is a primary phenomenon or a downstream effect of the affective storm characterizing this disorder.

Silk and colleagues in Chapter 5 also explore the linkage between anxiety/panic disorders and similar phenomena in BPD. Instead of using peripheral markers, these researchers report on the provocation of clinical anxiety/panic states using a lactate infusion. This pharmacological challenge approach has the potential for identifying specific provocative stimuli operating through specific biological mechanisms, linking phenomena with underlying biology. However, several caveats must be issued before venturing across such a "pharmacological bridge." The sensitivity and specificity of a particular pharmacological stimulus may be limited: a given stimulus may not consistently produce the target state, and a variety of stimuli using different target mechanisms may produce similar clinical states. The resultant state may differ in subtle (but possibly informative) ways from the naturally occurring state. Silk et al. have appropriately addressed these limitations, while presenting a sophisticated approach to BPD phenomenology and biology.

Evidence linking the serotonergic system with disorders of impulse control was described previously. DeVegvar et al. in Chapter 2 report on the application of pharmacological probes of the serotonergic system with neuroendocrine output measures. They find that blunted prolactin (PRL) responses to a fenfluramine challenge are associated with impulsive/aggressive behavioral patterns, both within and across diagnoses. This chapter is particularly noteworthy for its elaboration of a dimensional model of a particular behavior that cuts across traditional diagnostic boundaries. It raises a number of provocative questions. Is impulsive/aggressive behavior a biologically separable dimension of psychopathology? Is the abnormality linked to impulsivity or to aggression, two potentially separable dimensions? Is the abnormality in the serotonergic system causal or is it permissive, requiring other biological, psychological, and/or social factors before it expresses itself in behavior?

As noted above, Siever and his group have made substantial conceptual and empirical contributions to the biology of dimensional psychopathology. The dimensional approach of this team is also evident in Chapter 3, in which Steinberg et al. report on pharmacological probes of the adrenergic and cholinergic systems. Basal norepinephrine is found to be correlated with impulsivity and risk taking, and the growth hormone response to clonidine is found to be correlated with irritability and risk taking. Early findings regarding the use of physostigmine as a pharmacological probe for dysphoric states are also presented, evoking the same complex questions about pharmacological probes noted above. Insofar as these neurotransmitter systems are linked to drive state and reward, these findings raise the difficult question of the relationship of the underlying drive state of the organism to emitted behavior. Does impulsive or aggressive behavior require both an elevated drive state and a permissive factor (perhaps in part serotonergic)? What is the relationship of adrenergic and cholinergic abnormalities to serotonergic abnormalities? The fundamental potential advantage of this group's approach will ultimately be the opportunity to develop a theory of the complicated interactions among these regulatory systems—the next step beyond the one neurotransmitter–one behavioral dimension correlations.

Finally, in Chapter 6 Goyer and colleagues provide a review of the limited literature on structural and functional brain imaging in BPD. In general, BPD has not been found to be associated with structural changes in the brain, although one study suggests that schizotypal personality disorder may demonstrate a degree of ventricular enlargement similar to that observed in schizophrenia. The only study of functional brain imaging in patients with BPD included patients with other personality disorders. It found an inverse correlation in the total group between lifetime history of violence and the global rate of cerebral glucose metabolism as well as the metabolic rate in several orbital frontal regions of interest. Thus, low metabolic rates in frontal regions were associated with more lifetime violence, an intriguing association in view of the various executive functions of the frontal lobe. In view of the number of planes and regions of interest examined, such exploratory studies require replication; however, these studies nonetheless suggest the value of a dimensional approach to the personality disorders—in this case, correlating a dimension of pathological behavior with functional activity in specific regions of the human brain.

FUTURE DIRECTIONS

This volume presents many of the current cutting edges of research into the biological components of the personality disorders. Perhaps equally importantly, it suggests the likely future directions of these research efforts.

Part of the effort will involve an attempt to define more clearly the clinical phenomena occurring in various personality disorders, defining similarities to and differences from analogous Axis I disorders in terms of both the phenomenology itself and the possible underlying biological abnormalities. Identification of "meaningful" subgroups within the existing personality disorders may facilitate the search for biological underpinnings. However, it is increasingly likely that "meaningful" subgroups can be obtained only through a wholesale rethinking of our nosology.

An elaboration of the dimensional approach to psychopathology and biology will be a prominent part of the next decade of research. There will certainly be further efforts to identify common psychopathological dimensions across "different" disorders. Research is also likely to focus on an integrated exploration of specific clinical phenomena across diagnoses (such as affective lability/reactivity, dysphoric states, and impulsivity/behavioral dyscontrol). This integrated exploration will employ probes of multiple neurotransmitter systems in each patient to develop a better understanding of the complex interactions among these regulatory systems.

The development of high-technology imaging will allow "closer" approaches to relevant central pathways in order to complement the more distant peripheral markers now employed. The use of relatively specific receptor ligands will permit a more direct assessment of central receptor characteristics and possibly central turnover rates. Blood flow imaging with positron-emission tomography (PET), single photon emission computed tomography (SPECT), or new magnetic resonance imaging (MRI) techniques is likely to be employed to study functional states, and this imaging will grow ever more sophisticated through the development of a variety of provocative stimuli or challenge paradigms. Magnetoencephalography may develop to the point where electrical activity in specific deeper structures of the brain can be assessed.

The most daunting task will be the development of integrative theories of personality and its disorders. Such theories will need to encompass constitutional/temperamental predispositions, developmental factors, trauma and the determinants of the psychological response to trauma, and more subtle issues of upbringing and social training. These biological investigations form one crucial component of this long-term project.

REFERENCES

Akiskal HS, Yerevanian BI, Davis GC, et al: The nosologic status of borderline personality: clinical and polysomnographic study. Am J Psychiatry 142:192–198, 1985

Andrulonis PA, Glueck BC, Stroebel CF, et al: Organic brain dysfunction and the borderline syndrome. Psychiatr Clin North Am 4:47–66, 1981

Cloninger CR: A systematic method for clinical description and classification of personality variants: a proposal. Arch Gen Psychiatry 44:573–588, 1987

Coccaro EF, Siever LJ, Owen KR, et al: Serotonin in mood and personality disorders, in Serotonin in Major Psychiatric Disorders. Edited by Coccaro EF, Murphy DL. Washington, DC, American Psychiatric Press, 1990, pp 71–97

Cowdry RW, Pickar D, Davies R: Symptoms and EEG findings in the borderline syndrome. Int J Psychiatry Med 15:201–211, 1985–1986

Gardner DL, Cowdry RW: Positive effects of carbamazepine on behavioral dyscontrol in borderline personality disorder. Am J Psychiatry 143:519–522, 1986

Gunderson JG, Phillips KA: A current view of the interface between borderline personality disorder and depression. Am J Psychiatry 148:967–975, 1991

Gunderson JG, Sabo AN: The phenomenological and conceptual interface between borderline personality disorder and PTSD. Am J Psychiatry 150:19–27, 1993

Herman JL, Perry JC, van der Kolk BA: Childhood trauma in borderline personality disorder. Am J Psychiatry 146:490–495, 1989

Kellner CH, Post RM, Putnam F, et al: Intravenous procaine as a probe of limbic system activity in psychiatric patients and normal controls. Biol Psychiatry 22:1107-1126, 1987

Kendler KS, Gruenberg AM, Strauss JS: An independent analysis of the Copenhagen sample of the Danish adoption study of schizophrenia, II: the relationship between schizotypal personality disorder and schizophrenia. Arch Gen Psychiatry 38:982–984, 1981

Lucas PB, Gardner DL, Wolkowitz OM, et al: Dysphoria associated with methylphenidate infusion in borderline personality disorder. Am J Psychiatry 144:1577–1579, 1987

Lucas PB, Gardner DL, Cowdry RW, et al: Cerebral structure in borderline personality disorder. Psychiatry Res 27:111–115, 1989

McNamara E, Reynolds CF III, Soloff PH, et al: EEG sleep evaluation of depression in borderline patients. Am J Psychiatry 141:182–186, 1984

Monroe RR: Episodic Behavioral Disorders. Cambridge, MA, Harvard University Press, 1970

Ogata SN, Silk KR, Goodrich S, et al: Childhood sexual and physical abuse in adult patients with borderline personality disorder. Am J Psychiatry 147:1008–1013, 1990

Russ MJ, Roth SD, Lerman A, et al: Pain perception in self-injurious patients with borderline personality disorder. Biol Psychiatry 32:501–511, 1992

Siever LJ: Biological markers in schizotypal personality disorder. Schizophr Bull 11:564–575, 1985

Siever LJ, Davis KL: A psychobiological perspective on the personality disorders. Am J Psychiatry 148:1647–1658, 1991

Siever LJ, Klar H, Coccaro EF: Psychobiologic substrates of personality, in Biologic Response Styles: Clinical Implications. Edited by Klar H, Siever LJ. Washington, DC, American Psychiatric Press, 1985, pp 37–66

Silk KR, Cohen R, Gold L, et al: Psychotic symptoms in borderline personality disorder: consideration for DSM-IV (abstract). Biol Psychiatry 25 (suppl 7A):88A, 1989

Snyder S, Pitts WM Jr: Electroencephalography of DSM-III borderline personality disorder. Acta Psychiatr Scand 69:129–134, 1984

Snyder S, Pitts WM Jr, Gustin Q: CT scans of patients with borderline personality disorder (letter). Am J Psychiatry 140:272, 1983

Teicher MH, Glod CA, Surrey J, et al: Childhood abuse and limbic system ratings in adult psychiatric outpatients. J Neuropsychiatry Clin Neurosci 5:301–306, 1993

van Reekum R, Conway C, Gansler D, et al: Neurobehavioral study of borderline personality disorder. J Psychiatry Neurosci 18:121–129, 1993

Westen D, Ludolph P, Misle B, et al: Physical and sexual abuse in adolescent girls with borderline personality disorder. Am J Orthopsychiatry 60:55–66, 1990

Widiger TA, Trull TJ, Hurt SW, et al: A multidimensional scaling of the DSM-III personality disorders. Arch Gen Psychiatry 44:557–563, 1987

Zanarini MC, Gunderson JG, Marino MF, et al: Childhood experiences of borderline patients. Compr Psychiatry 30:18–25, 1989

Zanarini MC, Gunderson JG, Frankenberg FR: Cognitive features of borderline personality disorder. Am J Psychiatry 147:57–63, 1990

Zweig-Frank H, Paris JF, Guzder J: Dissociation in female patients with BPD. Paper presented at the 146th annual meeting of the American Psychiatric Association, San Francisco, CA, May 22–27, 1993

Chapter 11

Implications of Biological Research for Clinical Work With Borderline Patients

Kenneth R. Silk, M.D.

The preceding chapters in this book have presented and reviewed a wide array of biological and neurobehavioral studies of borderline patients. While these studies represent sophisticated research approaches to exploring the biological underpinnings of borderline personality disorder, at times they seem very far from clinical reality. Most clinicians do not have the time, expertise, or facilities to evaluate borderline patients "biologically," and even if they did have both the personnel and the resources, clinicians would wonder how these biological studies impact upon the everyday clinical management of the borderline patient.

The word *management* should be emphasized, because it appears that borderline patients need management as much as they need other aspects of treatment. Management encompasses the entire clinical approach to and overview of the borderline patient. It seems that nothing that is done with borderline patients is simple. Prescribing medications to a borderline patient is a complicated process even when there are strong clinical indications that a particular medication might be quite useful in a given patient. The process of prescribing medication to the patient must be managed, whether that management involves coordinating the pharmacological treatment with the therapist who provides the dynamic, cognitive, or group therapy in order to avoid or at least to minimize splitting (Silk, in press); or, in the situation where the therapist and the prescriber are the same person, avoiding the pitfall of polypharmacy and minimizing the feeling in the patient that the therapist-turned-prescriber has abandoned the more intimate aspects of the psychotherapy for the safer, more distant perspective of the biological psychiatrist (Gunderson 1984, 1986; Kubie 1971). The process of successfully prescribing a medication to a borderline patient may have as much to do with the "process" of when and how the medication is introduced into the treatment as it has to do with the actual choice of the medication itself.

This statement is not meant to imply that words can counteract the effects of medications; it is merely to place forward for consideration the idea that the words used to present and discuss the medication may have as much influence on the outcome of the process of prescribing medication as the actual biological interaction of the medication and the patient. A borderline patient should be told at the beginning of treatment that the suggestion that she or he take medications may occur sometime during the course of the treatment, and that the decision to prescribe medication does not mean that the "talking" part of the treatment is failing or that the patient is getting worse (Waldinger and Frank 1989a, 1989b). Rather, as one gets to know a patient better, one may be able to appreciate more fully which of the many symptoms manifested by the patient can become "target" symptoms for psychopharmacological intervention. In the borderline patient, these target symptoms are the symptoms that can be dissected out and followed over some period of time apart from the rapidly changing affective states and recurrent interpersonal crises.

BORDERLINE PERSONALITY DISORDER AND DIMENSIONS OF PSYCHOPATHOLOGY

Attention has more recently focused on the neurological and biological underpinnings of some of the cardinal but nondepressive symptoms of BPD—more specifically, the cognitive distortions, the affective instability, the impulsivity (and anger as perhaps a manifestation of that impulsivity), and the anxiety (Siever and Davis 1991). These "second generation" (see the Introduction to this volume) biological and pharmacological studies, which took place primarily in the second half of the 1980s and the early 1990s, moved away from attempting to find the specific biological substrate that might be awry in a specific personality disorder; rather, they proceeded toward trying to determine which biological subsystem or subsystems may be most closely related to specific dimensions of personality. Cloninger (1987) proposed a system for classifying personality variants along three dimensions: behavioral activation or novelty seeking, behavioral inhibition or harm avoidance, and behavioral maintenance or reward dependence. Cloninger posited that each dimension was closely tied to a neurotransmitter system: dopamine to behavioral activation, serotonin to behavioral inhibition, and norepinephrine to behavioral maintenance.

Siever and Davis (1991) expanded on the idea of the relationship of dimensions of personality to biological indices. They suggested associations among specific dimensions of personality psychopathology, biological indices, and the three Axis II clusters, and presented four dimensions of personality psychopathology: 1) a cognitive perceptual dimension, which is the primary disturbance found in the odd cluster of personality disorders (schizotypal, schizoid, paranoid) and which may result from disturbances in the dopamine system; 2) an impulsivity/aggression dimension, which is a dominant disturbance in the dramatic cluster (histrionic, narcissistic, borderline, antisocial) and which may be closely tied to the serotonergic system (see Chapter 2); 3) an affective instability dimension, which is also an essential disturbance in the dramatic cluster and which may be closely tied to the cholinergic and noradrenergic systems (see Chapters 3 and 4); and 4) an anxiety inhibition dimension, which is strongly involved in the anxious cluster (avoidant, dependent, passive-aggressive, obsessive-compulsive) and which may have its underlying disturbance in an autonomic function that can be tested with probes such as sodium lactate and yohimbine (see Chapters 4 and 5).

Empirical research into the underlying biological processes in personality disorder patients as well as the specific responses of some borderline patients to pharmacological agents lend support to this strategy of pursuing dimensions of psychopathology rather than specific diagnoses to better understand the biology of personality disorders. Perhaps these dimensions may be areas of psychopathology that need to be more fully excavated and understood in each of our patients before pharmacological decisions are made. Rather than attempting to elucidate each and every DSM-III-R (American Psychiatric Association 1987) symptom in order to arrive at an Axis II diagnosis, there may be greater clinical utility in exploring each of the four dimensions more thoroughly, even though these dimensions cut across specific categorical diagnoses. More thorough clinical exploration of each of these dimensions may lead to an informed pharmacological choice, a choice based upon some putative biological substrate underlying the most prominent pathological dimension.

It is the biological studies of the latter three dimensions—the dimensions of impulse/aggression, affective instability, and anxiety inhibition or excitation—that have been presented in this book. As summarized in Chapter 2, the evidence for a relationship between aggression (and perhaps impulsivity) and serotonin has been growing. As early as 1976, Åsberg and her colleagues pointed out the relationship between low cerebrospinal fluid (CSF) 5-hydroxyindoleacetic acid (5-HIAA) and violence against the self, particularly as it pertains to suicide. Coccaro and his colleagues (1989) brought home the relationship between serotonin and impulsive aggression to the personality disorders. By employing an infusion study of the response of prolactin to infused fenfluramine, a 5-hydroxytryptamine (5-HT) releasing/uptake inhibiting agent, Coccaro et al. were able to show an inverse correlation between prolactin response and measures of impulsive aggression against self and others. This inverse relationship between prolactin and impulsive aggression occurred only among the personality disorder patients, not among the depressed control subjects, and 44% of the personality disorder patients in this cohort met criteria for BPD. This work provides us with important evidence linking a specific dimension of behavior among borderline and other personality disorder patients to a specific neurotransmitter system.

IMPLICATIONS FOR PHARMACOLOGICAL TREATMENT

There have been three recent studies indicating that fluoxetine, a selective serotonin reuptake inhibitor, may be an effective treatment for some of the impulsivity and aggressivity of borderline patients (Cornelius et al. 1990; Markovitz et al. 1991; Norden 1989). All three studies are open-labeled. If this specific behavioral response to fluoxetine can be shown to persist in more rigorously designed studies (i.e., double-blind, crossover studies that employ placebo control subjects), this method of exploring the specific biological underpinnings of a dimension of behavior and of prescribing a specific pharmacological agent to address that dimension may be a rewarding approach to the treatment of personality disorder patients.

Siever et al. (1992), in their studies of increased growth hormone response to intravenous clonidine in personality disorder patients, suggest a relationship between the noradrenergic system and risk taking, irritability, and impulsivity, all of which seem to culminate in an individual's having a heightened reactivity to the environment. Perhaps a heightened reactivity to the environment (modulated by the noradrenergic system) and an increased propensity to impulsive aggression (modulated by the serotonergic system) combine to form a particularly troublesome behavioral picture in borderline patients (see Chapter 2). This particular behavioral constellation may respond positively to the monoamine oxidase inhibitors (MAOIs), drugs that have been shown to be effective in some borderline patients (Cowdry and Gardner 1988; Leibowitz and Klein 1981; Leibowitz et al. 1984; Parsons et al. 1989; Soloff et al. 1993). MAOIs are thought to be particularly useful in hysteroid dysphoria patients, a group of patients who appear to act out self-destructively in response to environmental triggers, particularly separation, in contrast to the more "emotionally unstable" borderline patients, who seem more resistant to the MAOIs and perhaps more responsive to major tranquilizers and lithium (Parsons et al. 1989). The description of the environmentally hyperresponsive hysteroid dysphoria patient certainly captures the essence of one particular type of borderline patient. If these patients' emotional instability in response to the environment can be tempered through biological intervention, perhaps the impulsive/aggressive behavior, which may be the behavioral "end response" of the patient's reaction to the environment, may be decreased as well. Here, again, a specific pharmacological agent—an MAOI—is chosen as a way to modify a specific dimension of behavior—hyperreactivity to the environment—as opposed to trying to choose a specific medication to treat a specific diagnosis.

Treatment with lithium, which has been shown to increase postsynaptic serotonergic receptor activity (Linnoila et al. 1983), decreases aggression in borderline patients (Links et al. 1990) as well as in some patients with severe personality disorders (Shader et al. 1974). Further, if lithium also decreases catecholaminergic function (Linnoila et al. 1983), then perhaps lithium also decreases aggression because it reduces both reactivity to the environment and the propensity to aggressive behavior in susceptible individuals. Lithium has been shown to decrease emotional lability and to improve mood in emotionally unstable character disorder (Rifkin et al. 1972), a diagnosis applied to individuals whose instability seems to derive more from endogenous dysregulation than from environmental hyperreactivity (Parsons et al. 1989).

The purported relationship of heightened reactivity to the environment and catecholamines (as described in Chapter 3) suggests a role for the minor tranquilizers in BPD, although there is some controversy as to whether minor tranquilizers ultimately lead to consistent improvement or only to transient improvement with subsequent disinhibited behavior and aggression (Faltus 1984; Gardner and Cowdry 1985). Perhaps short-acting benzodiazepines such as alprazolam are more likely to lead to disinhibited behavior, since the patient experiences greater dysphoria associated with more rapidly decreasing blood levels, and longer-acting benzodiazepines may prove to be less disinhibiting in this regard. Although well-controlled pharmacological trials of benzodiazepines are needed in borderline patients, these treatments should be undertaken with caution because we run the risk of the patient's developing dependence on drugs like alprazolam (Green and Curtis 1988), particularly when this patient group has a significant propensity to abuse alcohol and other substances (Dulit et al. 1990).

Research by Siever and his colleagues (see Chapter 3) has revealed an increase in depressive response to physostigmine in borderline or "emotionally labile" patients when compared with other personality disorder patients. Perhaps the anticholinergic as well as the antidopaminergic effects of the neuroleptics can be useful in treating a "cholinergic-driven" depression (Soloff et al. 1986). Siever and colleagues make the argument for increased affective instability in cholinergic-sensitive individuals, and perhaps the predisposition toward affective lability—and, in particular, the "depressive lability" or sensitivity of borderline patients—may be closely related to the sensitivity of their cholinergic systems. As yet there is little evidence for a good pharmacological agent to treat the depressive reactivity or lability in borderline patients. Carbamazepine and lithium carbonate, mood stabilizers in "pure" (nonborderline) mood disorder patients, have been shown to be effective in borderline patients, but their effectiveness has been in controlling impulsivity rather than in maintaining mood stability. Cowdry and Gardner (1988) in their studies of carbamazepine, as well as Links et al. (1990) in their study of lithium, state specifically that the improvement in behavior did not appear to be the result of improved mood, and in fact may have led to more depression in Cowdry and Gardner's carbamazepine-treated cohort (Gardner and Cowdry 1986). However, the decrease in impulsivity may have been related to greater emotional stability rather than to improvement of mood, and patients reported decreased irritability and more time to think before they acted.

Borderline patients' hyperresponsivity to the environment and possible responsiveness to MAOIs and perhaps benzodiazepines, as well as these patients' propensity to self-medicate often with alcohol (Zanarini et al. 1991), lead one to scrutinize more closely the relationship of borderline patients to anxious patients. The recent rush of studies that reveal a high prevalence of childhood sexual abuse among borderline patients (Herman et al. 1989; Links et al. 1988; Ogata et al. 1990; Zanarini et al. 1989) and the possible relationship of borderline symptoms to post-abuse sequelae (Gunderson and Sabo 1993), as well as the argument that many borderline patients may actually be suffering from posttraumatic stress disorder (Herman and van der Kolk 1987), reinforce the possibility of a relationship between BPD and the anxiety disorders. Yehuda and colleagues, in a series of studies that are reviewed in Chapter 4, have explored the possible role of biogenic amines in borderline patients. Their studies reveal that borderline patients' biological responses within the catecholamine system appear very different from the responses of depressive patients. Our own preliminary work with sodium lactate, as elaborated in Chapter 5, suggests that some borderline patients seem to share a propensity for panic attacks or prolonged and uncomfortable states of heightened anxiety, but as with most symptoms and/or biological tests in borderline patients, the relationship between the patient's clinical complaint and the biological test result is unclear. If borderline patients suffer panic attacks, the attacks are atypical at best, since they seem to be in reaction to a specific environmental or psychological situation. Also, these panic attacks may last for hours, leading to a prolonged period of dissociation that may only eventually be relieved through some form of self-mutilation (Leibenluft et al. 1987). In other circumstances, the anxiety seems to build slowly over time until a near panic state is reached, followed by dissociation and then self-mutilation. This serves to calm the person, but only temporarily, and then the cycle of increased tension, panic, dissociation, and cutting repeats itself. Perhaps some of the positive response that some borderline patients have had to fluoxetine and the MAOIs relates to the ability of these medications to control panic, and this underlying propensity to panic may be behind much of the emotional instability found among some borderline patients. Benzodiazepines may have real benefit for these panic-prone borderline patients, and we need more studies to better understand whether alcohol abuse in some borderline patients serves an antipanic, anti-agoraphobic function.

IMPLICATIONS FOR CLINICAL EVALUATION

These biological studies reinforce the ideas of Siever and Davis (1991) as well as Cloninger (1987), that perhaps clinicians need to evaluate personality disorder patients along dimensions of behavior such as cognitive disturbance, impulsivity/aggression, emotional lability, and anxiety. This is not to say that we should adopt a dimensional classification system at this point; rather, we need to look more closely at which particular dimension(s) may be most disordered in any given borderline or personality disorder patient. Biological and pharmacological studies support exploration of the dimensions of impulsivity and aggressivity and treatment with serotonergic agents. When the aggression and impulsivity is confounded by hyperreactivity to the environment, we need to consider the noradrenergic system and perhaps pharmacological treatment with MAOIs. When the noradrenergic system dysfunction or dysregulation appears more directly related to early trauma, with guarded hyperalertness and expectation of malevolence from the world (Nigg et al. 1991), then perhaps the MAOIs or the serotonergic compounds or the benzodiazepines or the neuroleptics may be the drugs of choice.

Unfortunately, we cannot subject all borderline patients to these biological explorations in order to try to determine which neurotransmitter system seems most dysregulated in any given patient. Nonetheless, clinicians need to pay attention to the biological research, for it guides us toward the behavioral dimensions that we need to explore more fully in our patients. Although we lack the skills or ease to provide sophisticated biological screening to all our borderline patients, we do not lack the expertise to examine clinically all of our borderline patients on these dimensions.

CONCLUSIONS

The studies reported in this book represent early stages of research in these areas, and we are far from having any definitive answers. Although we have no clear biological answers, we nonetheless should not assume that everything is developmental and needs to be approached primarily through psychotherapy, a mode of treatment that has not proved to be greatly successful in borderline patients (Waldinger and Gunderson 1984). If psychotherapy is to be efficacious with borderline patients, we need to find pharmacological as well as psychological "holding environments" (Modell 1976) so that psychotherapeutic work can proceed more calmly and more constructively. This is not to imply that the treatment of BPD patients should be solely through biological means. These patients won't allow it—they demand great amounts of our time, and no matter how hard we try to avoid the transference issues, they nevertheless appear. Thus, we as clinicians need to pay attention to the relationship that exists between us and the borderline patient even if we choose a role as the patient's psychopharmacologist. However, choosing a role or treatment that pays less attention to transference/countertransference issues does not mean that these issues disappear (Beck and Freeman 1990).

While there is always too much transference (a major but unavoidable danger) in the treatment of borderline patients, there can also be too much medication. Whereas it may seem useful to treat a patient for disturbances in all dimensions simultaneously, there is no indication that polypharmacy is any more successful in patients with BPD than in other patients. Despite these first- and second-generation biological studies, the treatment of borderline patients, pharmacological or otherwise, remains empirical. Any pharmacological treatment should be tried over a period long enough to evaluate whether the behavioral dimension chosen for pharmacological intervention has actually changed in an improved direction. We need to be modest in our goals and look for a response in clearly defined but limited areas of symptomatology. If one medication does not lead to improvement in the defined, circumscribed area, that medication should be stopped, new dimensions or symptom targets determined, and a different medication, by itself, tried for a length of time sufficient to see a response.

Empirical treatment does not mean uninformed treatment. These studies inform us of possible dimensions in which disturbances can occur, and we need to empirically and clinically use this information to explore these dimensions in an attempt to provide more sophisticated treatment to our patients as we await further developments in the study of the biology of borderline personality disorder.

It would appear from these studies that BPD, despite operationalized diagnostic instruments, remains a heterogeneous disorder. However, at this juncture, that heterogeneity does not mean that we should abandon the diagnostic category. We may eventually use these biological dimensions to separate borderline patients into subgroups and to study those subgroups, particularly with respect to biological tests, pharmacological responsiveness, and relationship to Axis I disorders. But, at the moment, too homogeneous a research sample of borderline patients would not have much generalizability to the clinical population of borderline patients.

There is no "pure" borderline patient. The concept of behavioral dimensions, although it reinforces the idea of the heterogeneity of the diagnosis, appears to accurately reflect dimensions that support observed clinical reality. Further refinement of these concepts of dimensions of behavioral psychopathology and continued exploration of the biological underpinnings of these dimensions should eventually lead to a better understanding of and a more sophisticated pharmacological and behavioral approach to this complex group of patients.

REFERENCES

American Psychiatric Association: Diagnostic and Statistical Manual of Mental Disorders, 3rd Edition, Revised. Washington, DC, American Psychiatric Association, 1987

Åsberg M, Träskman L, Thorén P: 5-HIAA in the cerebrospinal fluid: a biochemical suicide predictor? Arch Gen Psychiatry 33:1193–1197, 1976

Beck AT, Freeman A: Cognitive Therapy of Personality Disorders. New York, Guilford, 1990

Cloninger CR: A systematic method for clinical description and classification of personality variants: a proposal. Arch Gen Psychiatry 44:573–588, 1987

Coccaro EF, Siever LJ, Klar HM, et al: Serotonergic studies in patients with affective and personality disorders: correlates with suicidal and impulsive aggressive behavior. Arch Gen Psychiatry 46:587–599, 1989

Cornelius JR, Soloff PH, Perel JM, et al: Fluoxetine trial in borderline personality disorder. Psychopharmacol Bull 26:151–154, 1990

Cowdry RW, Gardner DL: Pharmacotherapy of borderline personality disorder: alprazolam, carbamazepine, trifluoperazine and tranylcypromine. Arch Gen Psychiatry 45:111–119, 1988

Dulit RA, Fyer MR, Haas GL, et al: Substance use in borderline personality disorder. Am J Psychiatry 147:1002–1007, 1990

Faltus FJ: The positive effect of alprazolam in the treatment of three patients with borderline personality disorder. Am J Psychiatry 141:802–803, 1984

Gardner DL, Cowdry RW: Alprazolam-induced dyscontrol in borderline personality disorder. Am J Psychiatry 142:98–100, 1985

Gardner DL, Cowdry RW: Development of melancholia during carbamazepine treatment in borderline personality disorder. J Clin Psychopharmacol 6:236–239, 1986

Green MA, Curtis GC: Personality disorders in panic patients: response to termination of antipanic medication. Journal of Personality Disorders 2:303–314, 1988

Gunderson JG: Borderline Personality Disorder. Washington, DC, American Psychiatric Press, 1984

Gunderson JG: Pharmacotherapy for patients with borderline personality disorder. Arch Gen Psychiatry 43:698–700, 1986

Gunderson JG, Sabo AN: The phenomenological and conceptual interface between borderline personality disorder and PTSD. Am J Psychiatry 150:19–27, 1993

Herman JL, van der Kolk BA: Traumatic antecedents of borderline personality disorder, in Psychological Trauma. Edited by van der Kolk BA. Washington, DC, American Psychiatric Press, 1987, pp 111–126

Herman JL, Perry JC, van der Kolk BA: Childhood trauma in borderline personality disorder. Am J Psychiatry 146:490–495, 1989

Kubie LS: The retreat from patients: an unanticipated penalty of the full-time system. Arch Gen Psychiatry 24:98–106, 1971

Leibenluft E, Gardner DL, Cowdry RW: The inner experience of the borderline self-mutilator. Journal of Personality Disorders 1:317–324, 1987

Liebowitz MR, Klein DF: Interrelationship of hysteroid dysphoria and borderline personality disorder. Psychiatr Clin North Am 4:67–87, 1981

Liebowitz MR, Quitkin FM, Stewart JW, et al: Phenelzine v imipramine in atypical depression: a preliminary report. Arch Gen Psychiatry 41:669–677, 1984

Links PS, Steiner M, Offord DR, et al: Characteristics of borderline personality disorder: a Canadian study. Can J Psychiatry 33:336–340, 1988

Links PS, Steiner M, Boiago I, et al: Lithium therapy for borderline patients: preliminary findings. Journal of Personality Disorders 4:173–181, 1990

Linnoila M, Virkkunen M, Scheinin M, et al: Low cerebrospinal fluid 5-hydroxyindoleacetic acid concentration differentiates impulsive from nonimpulsive violent behavior. Life Sci 33:2609–2614, 1983

Markovitz PJ, Calabrese JR, Schulz SC, et al: Fluoxetine in the treatment of borderline and schizotypal personality disorders. Am J Psychiatry 148:1064–1067, 1991

Modell A: "The holding environment" and the therapeutic action of psychoanalysis. J Am Psychoanal Assoc 24:285–307, 1976

Nigg JT, Silk KR, Westen D, et al: Object representations in the early memories of sexually abused borderline patients. Am J Psychiatry 148:864–869, 1991

Norden MJ: Fluoxetine in borderline personality disorder. Prog Neuropsychopharmacol Biol Psychiatry 13:885–893, 1989

Ogata SN, Silk KR, Goodrich S, et al: Childhood sexual and physical abuse in adult patients with borderline personality disorder. Am J Psychiatry 147:1008–1013, 1990

Parsons B, Quitkin FM, McGrath PJ, et al: Phenelzine, imipramine, and placebo in borderline patients meeting criteria for atypical depression. Psychopharmacol Bull 25:524–534, 1989

Rifkin A, Quitkin F, Carillo C, et al: Lithium carbonate in emotionally unstable character disorder. Arch Gen Psychiatry 27:519–523, 1972

Shader RI, Jackson AH, Dodes LM: The anti-aggressive effects of lithium in man. Psychopharmacology 40:17–24, 1974

Siever LJ, Davis KL: A psychobiological perspective on the personality disorders. Am J Psychiatry 148:1647–1658, 1991

Siever LJ, Coccaro EF, Trestman RL, et al: The growth hormone response to clonidine in acute and remitted depressed male patients. Neuropsychopharmacology 6:165–177, 1992

Silk KR: Rational pharmacotherapy for personality disordered patients, in Personality Disorders: A Practical Guide to Clinical Management. Edited by Links P. Washington, DC, American Psychiatric Press, in press

Soloff PH, George A, Nathan RS, et al: Progress in the pharmacotherapy of borderline disorders. Arch Gen Psychiatry 43:691–697, 1986

Soloff PH, Cornelius J, George A, et al: Efficacy of phenelzine and haloperidol in borderline personality disorder. Arch Gen Psychiatry 50:377–385, 1993

Waldinger RJ, Frank AF: Clinicians' experiences in combining medication and psychotherapy in the treatment of borderline patients. Hosp Comm Psychiatry 40:712–717, 1989a

Waldinger RJ, Frank AF: Transference and the vicissitudes of medication use by borderline patients. Psychiatry 52:416–427, 1989b

Waldinger RJ, Gunderson JG: Completed psychotherapies with borderline patients. Am J Psychother 38:190–202, 1984

Zanarini MC, Gunderson JG, Marino MF, et al: Childhood experiences of borderline patients. Compr Psychiatry 30:18–25, 1989

Zanarini MC, Gunderson JG, Frankenburg FR, et al: Pathways to health for borderline patients. Paper presented at the 144th annual meeting of the American Psychiatric Association, New Orleans, LA, May 1991

Index

*Page numbers printed in **boldface** type refer to tables or figures.*

Acetylcholine, 44, 46, 48, 55
Acetylcholinesterase, **47**
Acetylcholinesterase
 inhibitors, 46
 depressive responses to,
  44–45
Adolescents
 CSF 5-HIAA concentrations,
  disruptive behavior
  and, 27
 neurological abnormalities,
  childhood abuse and,
  190–192, **193–195**
Affective disorders. *See* Mood
 disorders
Affective instability, 55
 in attention disorders, 130
 Axis II disorders and, 42
 in borderline personality
  disorder, 41, 55–56, 64,
  215
 cholinergic system and,
  49–51, 55
 cholinomimetic challenge
  study of, 50–51
 medications for, 53, 232
 noradrenergic system and,
  45, 53–54, 55
Affective Lability Scale (ALS),
 50
Aggression, 23. *See also*
 Impulsivity; Suicide
 cerebral blood flow and, 117
 cerebral glucose metabolism
  and, 115–116, 117, 118,
  119
 CSF 5-HIAA concentrations,
  and, 27, 32, 43
 EEG abnormalities, 184
 fluoxetine effect on, 24–26
 gender differences in, 33–34
 impulsive, 24, 35–36, 43, 231
  family study, 32–33
  fenfluramine and, 30–31,
   43, 230
  noradrenergic system
   role in, 32, 51
 limbic kindling and, 180, 182
 in organic brain damage, 35
 pharmacological treatment,
  35
 serotonergic function and,
  24–26, 30–33, 200, 231
 serotonin uptake and,
  28–29
 verbal, 34, 54
Alcohol abuse, in borderline
 personality disorder, 232,
 234
Alpha$_2$-adrenergic agonists,
 clonidine, 31–32, 52
Alpha$_2$-adrenergic receptor
 binding
 anxiety symptoms and, 76,
  78, 79–80
 benzodiazepines and, 75–80

Alpha$_2$-adrenergic receptor binding *(continued)*
  in borderline personality disorder, 74, 75–78, **77, 79**
  differences in borderline personality disorder and major depressive disorder, 63
  in major depressive disorder, 69–70, 71–73, **72, 73**
    with comorbid borderline personality disorder, **72**, 73–75, **73**
  norepinephrine release and, 74
Alpha$_2$-adrenergic receptors, 69
  functioning in major depression, 52
Alprazolam, 232
Amitriptyline, xxiii
Amygdala, 180, 183, 200
Anger, 4–5, 17, 19, 130, 213
Anticholinergics, behavioral effects, 47
Antidepressants, tricyclic, xxiii, 97
Antisocial personality disorder, 101, 168
  cerebral glucose metabolism in, 116–117
  comorbid borderline personality disorder prognosis and, 9
Anxiety
  and alpha$_2$-adrenergic receptor binding, 76, 78, 79–80
  in borderline personality disorder, 76, 78–79, 93, 96–97, 99, 103–104, 212
Anxiety disorders
  borderline personality disorder relationship to, 93–95, 212, 220, 234
  noradrenergic system and, 179
Arecoline, 46, **47**, 48
Atropine, 46, **47**
Attention-deficit disorder, 160, 216
Attention deficits, in borderline personality disorder, 129, 130
Attention-deficit hyperactivity disorder, 17, 130
  clonidine and, 52
  impulsivity and, 19
Auditory processing, in borderline personality disorder, 144–145
Axis I disorders, 42. *See also specific disorders*
  biological abnormalities in, 42
  borderline personality disorder relationship to, 210–212
Axis II disorders. *See* Personality disorders; *specific disorders*

Barratt Impulsivity Scale (BIS), 5, 12

Diagnostic Interview for
Borderlines correlation,
14, 15–16, **15**
motor behavior subscale, 30,
53
risk-taking subscale, 54
Benzodiazepines, 75–76, **77**,
78, **79**, 232, 233, 234, 235
alpha$_2$-adrenergic receptor
binding and, 75–80, **77**,
79
effect on depression, 76
Bipolar disorder, 48
Block Span/Corsi Blocks test,
136–137, 138, 139, 141, 142
Blood flow imaging, 222
Borderline personality
disorder, 23, 177
behavior dimensional
classification for, 235,
237
clinical features, xvii–xviii,
64
concepts of, xviii–xxi, 64,
91–92, 159–161
diagnosis, xviii–xxi, 23, 110
MAO activity and, 68–69, **68**
neurodevelopmental
factors, 161
prognosis, 8–9
symptoms, 23, 64, 96
Boredom, 64
Brain. *See also* Organic brain
abnormalities
amygdala, 180, 183, 200
blood flow, 115, 117
development, 182–183
childhood abuse effects
on, 183–185

hemispheric asymmetry,
childhood abuse and,
195, 196–197, 199
hemispheric integration,
182, 200
hemispheric specialization,
181
hippocampus, 179, 183
5-HT$_2$ receptor binding, **25**,
26
imipramine receptor
binding, **25**
lesions, 17, 129, 180–181
limbic system, 179
locus coeruleus, 51, 179
prefrontal cortex, 180–181,
200
development, 182–183
dopamine projections,
182–183
probe auditory evoked
potential attenuation,
197–199
right hemisphere
emotion and, 181–182, 197
painful memories and,
197–199
trauma and, 197–199
structural abnormalities, 170
temporal lobe dysfunction,
173
ventricular size
in borderline personality
disorder, 111–112,
114, 118, 129, 162, 170
in schizophrenia, 110, 111
in schizotypal
personality disorder,
110, 111, 114, 118

Brain electrical mapping
(BEAM), 190, 191, 218
Brain imaging, 222–223
of borderline personality
disorder, 162, **166**, **167**,
170, 216, 221
of childhood abuse patients,
190, **193**
functional imaging,
114–118, 119
of personality disorders,
166, **167**
positron-emission
tomography (PET),
114–115
of psychiatric disorders,
109, 111–112, 119,
166–168, **166**, **167**
single photon emission
computed tomography
(SPECT), 115
structural imaging, 112–113,
119
Brief Psychiatric Rating Scale
(BPRS), 114
Brown-Goodwin Assessment
for Life History of
Aggression (BGA), 5
Buspirone
personality disorders and, 33
as serotonin index, **25**, 33
Buss-Durkee Hostility
Inventory (BDHI), 4, 5, 12
assault subscale, 30, 53
Diagnostic Interview for
Borderlines correlation,
13–14, **13**, **15**
irritability subscale, 7, 30,
32, 33

Carbamazepine, 1, 6, 53, 233
Catecholamine metabolism,
219–220, 234
in borderline personality
disorder vs major
depressive disorder, 63,
66–80, 80
in chronic stress disorders,
74–75
Central nervous system
dysfunction. *See*
Neurological
dysfunction
Cerebrospinal fluid (CSF)
5-HIAA concentrations
aggression and, 26–27,
32, 43
fenfluramine and, 32, 43
in personality disorders,
31–32
as serotonin index, **25**, 28,
36
suicidality and, 6, 27–28,
29
3-methoxy-4-hydroxy-
phenylglycol (MHPG)
concentrations, 52
Childhood abuse
in borderline personality
disorder, 64, 80, 178,
212–213
brain development effects
of, 183–185, 200
brain hemispheric
asymmetry and, **195**,
196–197, 199
EEG abnormalities and, 184,
190, 192, **193–195**,
196–197

gender differences, 189–190, **189**
limbic kindling and, 180, 200
limbic system dysfunction and, 187–190, **189**
  age differences, 188–189
  gender differences, 189–190
neurocognitive functioning and, 148
neurological assessments of, 191–192, **193**
neurological dysfunction and, 168–170, **169**
psychological abuse, 196, 197
psychological effects of, 177–178
sexual abuse, 168–169, **169**, 188, 188–190, **189**
therapy, in adulthood, 200–201
Children
  abused, neurological abnormalities, 190–192, **193–195**
  attention disorders in, 130
  CSF 5-HIAA concentrations, disruptive behavior and, 27
  response to clonidine, in attention-deficit hyperactivity disorder, 52
m-Chlorophenylpiperazine, as serotonin index, **25**, 34
Cholinergic agonists, 46, **47**, 48

Cholinergic system
  affective instability and, 49–51, 55
  depression and, 44–45
  dysphoria and, 43
  mood disorders and, 44–45, 46–49
  neuroendocrine challenge tests, 46–47, **47**
  REM sleep latency and, 45
Cholinomimetics
  behavioral effects, 46
  sleep effects, 48
Clonidine, 31–32, 80, 231
  attention-deficit hyperactivity disorder and, 52
  borderline personality disorder and, 53–54
  depression and, 52
  growth hormone response to, 31–32, 52, 54
  irritability and, 31–32
  in obsessive-compulsive disorder, 52
  in panic disorder, 52
  personality disorders and, 54
  in schizophrenia, 52
  suicidality and, 32
Clozapine, xviii
Cognitive dysfunction. *See also* Memory impairment; Visuospatial processing
  affective dysregulation and, 149
  in borderline personality disorder, 127–128, 131–132, 186, 217–218

Cognitive dysfunction
   (continued)
   organic basis for, 147–150
   verbal skills, 144
   childhood abuse and, 148
   dissociation and, 148–149
   in personality disorders, 186
Computed tomography (CT). *See* Brain imaging
Continuous Performance Task, **136**
Corsi Blocks/Block Span test, **136–137**, 138, 139, 141, 142
CSF. *See* Cerebrospinal fluid
Cyclothymia, 101

Delayed Memory of Three Word Pairs, **136**, 142, 143, 145
Depersonalization, 98
Depression. *See also* Major depressive disorder
   biological abnormalities in, 44
   cholinergic sensitivity in, 44–45, 48–49
   noradrenergic hyporesponsivity in, 45, 51–52
   norepinephrine metabolites production in, 52
   REM sleep latency in, 45
   serotonergic function and, 30
Dexamethasone suppression test, xxi, xxii, 66, 110, 211
Diagnosis
   of affective disorder, 96
   of borderline personality disorder, 23, 110, 229–230
   borderline personality disorder, "disturbed Rorschach–intact WAIS," 129, 132, 134
   of borderline personality disorder, historical evolution, xviii–xxi
   borderline vs schizotypal personality disorder, 128
   of panic disorder, 103
Diagnostic Interview for Borderlines (DIB), xxi, 3, 8, 9, 11, 71, 95, 109, 164
   Barratt Impulsivity Scale correlation, **14**, 15–16, **15**
   Buss-Durkee Hostility Inventory correlation, 13–14, **13**, **15**
   as impulsivity measure, 16
   Suicidal Behaviors Questionnaire correlation, 14–15, **14**, **15**
Diagnostic Interview for Personality Disorders (DIPD), 164
Dialectical behavior therapy (DBT)
Diisopropylfluorophosphate (DFP), 46, **47**
Dissociation
   in borderline personality disorder, 97, 98, 213
   EEG abnormalities and, 184–185
   neurocognitive functioning and, 148–149

Dissociative Experience Scale (DES), 187
Dopamine, prefrontal cortex development and, 182–183
Dysphoria, cholinergic sensitivity and, 43
Dysthymia, 95, 97, 101

Eating disorders, 213
EEG abnormalities, 218. *See also* Neurological dysfunction
 in borderline personality disorder, 129, 161–162, 167, 186
 childhood abuse and, 184, 190, 192, 196–197
  age differences, **193**
  gender differences, **193**
  hemispheric localization, **195**, 196–197
  regional localization, 192, **194**
 dissociation and, 184–185
 in multiple personality disorder, 184–185
 in personality disorders, 167
 in temporal lobe epilepsy, 184–185
 violent behavior and, 184
Embedded Figures Test, **137**, 139, 142, 145, 147
Emotion
 neural regulation of, 182
 right hemisphere role in, 181–182
Environmental sensitivity
 in borderline personality disorder, 41, 231
 noradrenergic system and, 43, 51, 52, 54, 231
Epilepsy, multiple personality disorder and, 184–185
Eye tracking, in schizotypy and schizophrenia, 110

Facial Memory Test, 144, 145
Fenfluramine
 borderline personality disorder and, 30–31
 CSF 5-HIAA concentrations and, 32, 43
 impulsivity and, 5
 personality disorders and, 30–31
 as serotonin index, 5, **25**, 29–30, 43
Finger Tapping Test, 140
Flashbacks, 102
18-Fluorodeoxyglucose, 115
Fluoxetine, 231
 aggression and, 24–26
 impulsivity reduced by, 35

Gamblers, 45, 52. *See also* Risk taking
Gender differences
 in aggression, 33–34
 in borderline personality disorder, 160
 in childhood abuse, 189–190, **189**
 EEG abnormalities, **193**
 limbic system dysfunction, 189–190
 serotonergic system, 34
Global Assessment Scale (GAS), 11, 14

Glucose metabolism (cerebral)
  aggression and, 115–116, 117, 118
  in antisocial personality disorder, 116–117
  in borderline personality disorder, 116
  impulsivity and, 119
  in obsessive-compulsive disorder, 114, 117–118
  in psychiatric disorders, 114–118
  substance abuse and, 114
Grooved Pegboard Test, 140

Haloperidol, xxiii
Hamilton Rating Scale for Depression (HRSD), xxiii, 29, 68, 75, 98
  benzodiazepine treatment and, 76
Head trauma, 166, **166**, **167**, 171
5-HIAA. *See* 5-Hydroxyindoleacetic acid
Hippocampus, 179, 183
Homovanillic acid (HVA), in schizotypy and schizophrenia, 110
Hopkins Symptom Checklist—90 (SCL-90), 6, 98, 187
5-HT$_2$ receptors, **25**
  suicide and, 26, 29
5-HT. *See* Serotonin
5-Hydroxyindoleacetic acid (5-HIAA)
  aggression and, 26–27, 32

fenfluramine and, 32, 43
in personality disorders, 31–32
as serotonin index, **25**, 28, 36, 215
suicidality and, 27–28, 29
5-Hydroxytryptamine (5-HT). *See* Serotonin
Hysteroid dysphoria, MAOI treatment, 45, 53, 231

Imipramine receptor binding, **25**
Impulsive aggression. *See under* Aggression
Impulsivity, 2–3, 23, 218. *See also* Aggression; Irritability
  anger element in, 4–5, 17, 19
  in antisocial personality disorder, 43
  attention-deficit hyperactivity disorder and, 19
  in attention disorders, 130
  in borderline personality disorder, 1–2, 18–19, 35–36, 43
  borderline personality disorder prognosis and, 8–9
  cerebral glucose metabolism and, 119
  correlations of various measures of, 12–16, **13**, **14**, **15**
  MAO activity and, 67
  noradrenergic system role in, 32
  norepinephrine and, 32, 54

in organic brain damage, 36
serotonergic activity and, 5, 18, 112, 119, 214–215, 220
suicidality and, 19
Incest. *See* Childhood abuse
Information processing impairments, in schizotypy and schizophrenia, 110
Instability (of mood). *See* Affective instability
Intelligence, in borderline personality disorder, 128
Irritability. *See also* Impulsivity
in borderline personality disorder, 4, 7, 17, 19, 53
noradrenergic system role in, 32, 45, 51, 53, 55
serotonergic system and, 5, 18

Kindling, 172, 180, 182, 200, 201

Lactate infusion. *See* Sodium lactate infusion
Learning disabilities, 130
Lesions
 brain, 17, 129
 prefrontal cortex, 180–181
 of serotonergic system, 24
Life Experience Questionnaire (LEQ), 188
Limbic system, 179
 childhood abuse influence on, 172, 187–190, **189**
 kindling, 172, 180, 182, 200, 201
 limbic striatum, 180

trauma and, 182, 215
Limbic System Checklist—33 (LSCL-33), 187, **189**, 190, 218
Lithium, 35, 67, 231, 232, 233
Lithium carbonate, 48, 53, 233
Locus coeruleus, 51, 74, 179
Longitudinal Expert Evaluation using all Data (LEAD), 95

McGlashan's Total Follow-Up Period Outcome Dimensions, 8
Magnetic resonance imaging (MRI). *See* Brain imaging
Major depressive disorder. *See also* Depression
 alpha$_2$-adrenergic receptor binding, 69–70, **72**, **73**
 borderline personality disorder relationship, 63, 65–66, 95
 borderline personality disorder as variant of, 64–65, 80
 cholinergic sensitivity in, 44
Management. *See* Patient management
MAO, in major depressive disorder, 67
MAO inhibitors, 45, 53, 97, 103, 231, 232, 233, 235
MAO (platelet)
 in borderline personality disorder, 67–69, **68**
 in borderline personality disorder vs major depressive disorder, 63

MAO (platelet) *(continued)*
  in major depressive
    disorder, 67
  personality characteristics
    influenced by, 67
Medications. *See also specific
  medications*
  for affective instability, 53
  benzodiazepines, 75–76,
    75–80, **77**, 78, **79**
  beta-blockers, 35
  MAO inhibitors, 45, 53, 97,
    103
  neuroleptics, xxiii
  serotonergic compounds,
    235
  to reduce aggression, 35
  tranquilizers, 231, 232
  tricyclic antidepressants,
    xxiii, 97
Memory, right brain
  hemisphere and, 197–199
Memory impairment, 128,
  131, **136–137**, 146–147. *See
  also* Cognitive dysfunction
  verbal memory, 142, 144–145
  visual memory, 141–142,
    144
3-Methoxy-4-hydroxy-
  phenylglycol (MHPG), 52
Methylphenidate, 52, 215
Minnesota Multiphasic
  Personality Inventory
  (MMPI), 27
Modified Aggression Scale
  (MAS), 117
Mood disorders
  affective instability in, 41,
    43, 56

biological abnormalities in,
  44
borderline personality
  disorder relationship to,
  xxii, 110–111
cholinergic sensitivity in,
  44–45, 46–49
cholinomimetics and,
  48–49
diagnosis, 96
physostigmine sensitivity
  in, 48
Mood instability. *See* Affective
  instability
Multiple personality disorder
  borderline personality
    disorder and, 213
  EEG abnormalities in,
    184–185
  temporal lobe epilepsy and,
    184–185
  trauma and, 212
Murderers
  cerebral glucose metabolism
    in, 116–117
  CSF 5-HIAA in, 27
Muscarinic agonists, 46, **47**
  cholinergic availability and,
    46, **47**
  depressive responses to,
    44–45
Muscarinic antagonists, 46, **47**
  cholinergic availability and,
    46, **47**

Neuroendocrine challenge
  tests
  in cholinergic system,
    46–47, **47**

in noradrenergic system, 31
to assess serotonergic functioning, **25**, 29–33
Neuroimaging. *See* Brain imaging
Neuroleptics, xxiii, 212, 233, 235
Neurological assessment
of borderline personality disorder, 163–169, **166**, **167**, 218–219
of childhood abuse, 191–192, **193**
of personality disorders, 166–169, **166**, **167**
soft signs, 163, 171
Neurological dysfunction. *See also* EEG abnormalities
in borderline personality disorder, 169, 185–186
childhood abuse and, 168–170, **169**
Neuropsychological studies
of borderline personality disorder, **143**, 150–151
test performance factors, 145–146
Neuropsychological tests. *See specific tests*
Neurotransmitter systems, affective instability and, 43
Neurotransmitters. *See specific neurotransmitters*
Noradrenergic system, 45
anxiety disorders and, 179
borderline personality disorder and, 54, 235
environmental sensitivity and, 43, 51, 52, 54, 231
hyperactivity, in risk takers, 45
hyporesponsivity, in depression, 45, 51–52
influence on hippocampus, 179
irritability and, 45, 51, 54, 55
locus coeruleus, 51
in mood disorders, 51–52
neuroendocrine challenge tests, 31, 54
role in impulsive/aggressive behaviors, 32
Norepinephrine
alpha$_2$-adrenergic receptor binding, receptor binding sites and, 74
impulsivity and, 54, 221
risk taking and, 32, 52, 221
trauma and, 182
Normetanephrine, 52

Obsessive-compulsive disorder
cerebral glucose metabolism in, 114, 117–118
clonidine response in, 52
serotonergic function in, 27, 34
Organic brain abnormalities, 35, 111. *See also* Brain
Oxotremorine, 46, **47**

Panic attacks, 74, 98, 212, 217, 234
induced by sodium lactate, 99, 101–102

Panic disorder, 96
  alpha$_2$-adrenergic receptor binding in, 99
  brain imaging studies, 114, 119
  clonidine response in, 52
  diagnosis, 103
Paranoia, 103
Patient management, 227–228
Personality, neural regulation of, 182, 229
Personality Diagnostic Questionnaire (PDQ), 95
Personality disorders
  brain imaging assessments, 166–168, **166**, **167**
  clonidine and, 54
  EEG abnormalities, 167, **167**
  5-hydroxyindoleacetic acid in, 31–32
  neurocognitive performance in, 186
  neurological assessments of, **166**
  rejection sensitivity in, 43
  theories of, 209–210
Personality Disorders Examination (PDE), 113
Physostigmine, 45, 46, **47**, 55, 233
  in mood disorders, 48
  mood response study, 50–51
Pindolol, 33
Platelets
  5-HT$_2$ receptor binding, **25**, 29
  imipramine receptor binding, **25**, 28–29
  MAO activity, 67
  serotonin uptake, **25**, 28–29

Positron-emission tomography (PET), 114–115
Posttraumatic stress disorder (PTSD), 80
  alpha$_2$-adrenergic receptor binding in, 99
  borderline personality disorder and, 63–64, 80
  borderline personality disorder relationship to, 94, 212–213
  cerebral glucose metabolism in, 114
  flashbacks, 102
PRL. *See* Prolactin
Probe auditory evoked potentials, 197–199
Procaine, 215
Profile of Mood States (POMS), 50, 198
Prolactin (PRL)
  irritability and, 5
  response to buspirone, 33
  response to fenfluramine, 5, **25**, 29–31, 43
    CSF 5-HIAA concentrations and, 32, 43
Propranolol, 35
Psychiatric disorders
  Axis I disorders, 42
  brain imaging of, 109, 111–112, 119
Psychological tests. *See* Neuropsychological tests; *specific tests*
Psychopathology, MAO activity and, 67

Psychotic episodes, in borderline personality disorder, 97, 217
Psychiatric disorders, cerebral glucose metabolism in, 114–115

Rage, 4–5, 17, 19, 130, 213
Rats, bred for cholinergic supersensitivity, 47
3H-Rauwolscine, 70
Rejection sensitivity, 43–44, 56
Research Diagnostic Criteria (RDC), 71, 75, 95, 96
Respiridone, xviii
Retrospective Family Pathology Questionnaire, 164–165
Rey-Osterrieth figure, **136–137**, 138–139, 140, 141, 145
Right brain hemisphere emotion and, 181–182, 197
trauma and, 197–199
Risk taking, 45, 54. *See also* Gamblers
Road-Map Test of Direction Sense, **137**, 139, 141
Rorschach test, 128
borderline personality disorder responses, 132–133
and WAIS, in borderline personality disorder, 129, 132, 134
RS86, 46, **47**, 48
Ruff Figural Fluency Test, **136**, 139, 140

SADS. *See* Schedule for Affective Disorders and Schizophrenia
Schedule for Affective Disorders and Schizophrenia (SADS), 50, 53, 71, 75, 96, 113
Schizophrenia, 209
biological abnormalities in, 42
borderline personality disorder similarities, xix, 211
brain imaging studies of, 111, 114
clonidine response in, 52
homovanillic acid levels in, 110
neurodevelopmental history, 161
schizotypal personality disorder compared, 42
serotonin uptake in, 28
Schizotypal personality disorder, 101, 211
diagnosis, 110
homovanillic acid levels in, 110
schizophrenia compared, 42
ventricular size in, 114
Scopolamine, 46, **47**
Seashore Rhythm Test, 145
Seashore Test of Tonal Memory, 145
Seasonal affective disorder, cerebral glucose metabolism in, 114
Seizures, 166, **166**, **167**, 168, 171, 215

Selective Reminding Test, **136**
Self-esteem, 56
Self-mutilation, 103, 216–217, 234
Sensation seeking, MAO activity and, 67
Serotonergic system abnormalities
    family histories of, 32–33
    impulsive aggression and, 35, 43, 112
    aggression and, 24–26, 30–33, 200
    depression and, 30
    gender differences in, 33–34
    impulsivity and, 5, 18, 112, 119
    lesions, 24
Serotonin (5-HT), 24
    binding studies, **25**
    indices, **25**
    metabolites, **25**
    neuroendocrine challenge tests, **25**, 29–33, 36
    suicide and, 26, 34
Sexton, Anne, 150
SIDP. *See* Structured Interview for DSM-III Personality Disorders
Single photon emission computed tomography (SPECT), 115, 222
Sleep
    cholinomimetics' effects on, 48–49
    REM latency, xxi, xxii–xxiii, 45, 48, 66, 111

Social Adjustment Scale—Self-Report (SAS-SR), 12, **15**, 18
Sodium lactate infusion, 99, 234
    in borderline personality disorder, 100–104, 220
    flashbacks from, 102
    response symptoms, 101–102
SPECT. *See* Single photon emission computed tomography
Street Gestalt Completion Test, 144
Stress, prefrontal cortex development and, 183
Stress disorders (chronic), catecholamine disturbances in, 74–75
Structured Clinical Interview for DSM-III-R Axis II Personality Disorders (SCID-II), 95
Structured Interview for DSM-III Personality Disorders (SIDP), 3–4, 50, 53, 94–95
Substance abuse, 214, 232, 234
    borderline personality disorder prognosis and, 9
    cerebral glucose metabolism in, 114
    MAO activity and, 67
    suicidality and, 8
Suicidal Behaviors Questionnaire (SBQ), 11–12

Diagnostic Interview for
Borderlines correlation,
14–15, **14, 15**
Suicidality
5-HT_2 receptors and, 29
in borderline personality
disorder, 23, 64, 97–98,
213
borderline personality
disorder prognosis and,
9
CSF 5-HIAA concentrations
and, 27–28, 29
clonidine and, 32
EEG abnormalities and, 184
imipramine receptor
binding and, 28–29
impulsivity and, 19
MAO activity and, 67
substance abuse and, 8
Suicide. *See also* Aggression
5-HT_2 receptors and, 26, 29
serotonin role in, 26, 34
Symptoms, of borderline
personality disorder, 23,
64, 96, 235

Temporal lobe dysfunction,
173
Therapy. *See also* Medications
for adults abused in
childhood, 200–201
dialectical behavior therapy, 1
patient management,
227–228
pharmacological, xviii, xxiii,
97, 228, 231–235, 236
psychoeducational
techniques, 149–150
transference issues, 236
Three Word Pairs, **136**, 142,
143, 145
Thyroid challenge studies, of
borderline personality
disorder, xxi, 111
Thyrotropin-releasing
hormone (TRH) test, xxi,
66, 211
Trail Making Test, **136**, 139,
140
Tranquilizers, 231, 232
Transference, in borderline
personality disorder, 236
Tranylcypromine, 6
Trauma, 212
limbic system and, 182, 215
norepinephrine and, 182
right brain hemisphere and,
197–199
Treatment. *See* Therapy
2 and 7 Test of Selection and
Sustained Attention, 140
Tyrosine, 51

Vanillylmandelic acid (VMA),
52
Verbal Incidental Learning
Test, 145
Verbal skills, borderline
personality disorder, 142,
144–145
Violence. *See* Aggression
Visual Search and Neglect
Test, **137**, 140
Visuospatial processing, in
borderline personality
disorder, 128, 135,
136–137, 138–141, 144

WAIS-R. *See* Wechsler Adult Intelligence Scale
Ward Scale of Impulse Action Patterns, 7
Wechsler Adult Intelligence Scale (WAIS), 128, **136–137**
 Block Design subtest, 138
 Digit Symbol subtest, 135–136, 138, 140, 141
 Object Assembly subtest, 144
 performance tests, 140
 and Rorschach test, in borderline personality disorder, 129, 132, 134
 thought disorder assessment by, 134
Wechsler Memory Scale (WMS)
 Associate Learning subtest, 142
 Logical Memory subtest, **136–137**, 142, 145
 Visual Reproduction subtest, **136–137**, 139, 141, 145
Wisconsin Card Sorting Test, 144
Women. *See* Gender differences

Yohimbine, 80